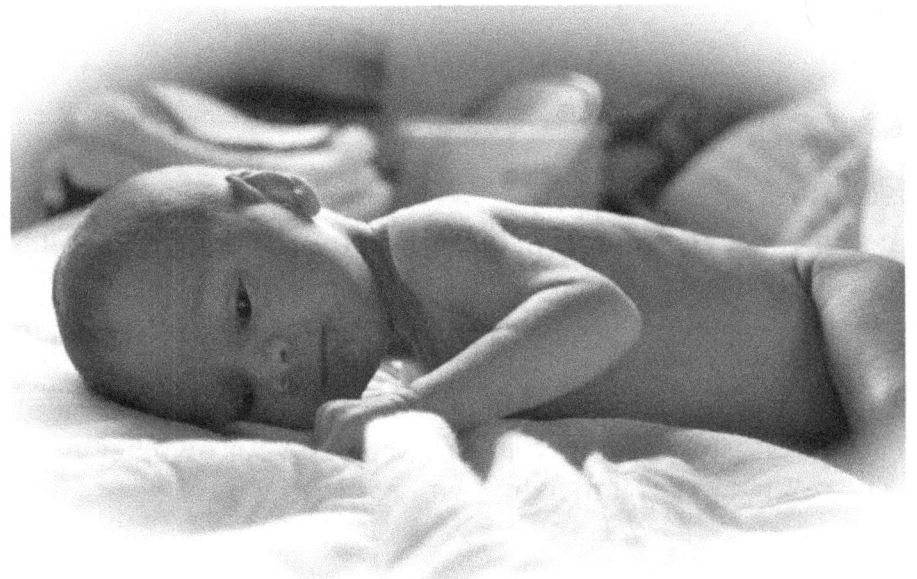

I dedicate this book to our beautiful little daughter,
Oria Berry Monarch, who lights up our lives.

Thank you for coming to join us;
we love you :)

Medical Disclaimer

This book is not intended to provide medical advice. All content, including text, graphics, images and information available in this book are for general informational and educational purposes only. The content is not intended to be a substitute for professional diagnosis or treatment. The author and publishers of this book are not responsible for any adverse effects that may occur from the application of the information in this book. You are encouraged to make your own healthcare decisions, based on your research and in partnership with a qualified healthcare professional.

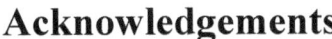

Acknowledgements

Huge gratitude to my wonderful partner in this game, Mr. Matt Monarch – thank you for all of your support, clarity and love, Bubba :)

To our beautiful little Oria Berry – thank you for coming here to join us; without you, this book would surely not exist.

Lotus blossoms of appreciation too to all the amazing women who have walked this path of childbearing before me – your strength is remarkable; thank you for all of the wisdom you share.

Infinite thanks to YOU too, dear reader, for having the courage to read this material – may you draw strength from the concepts shared here, to co-create a gentle start for your own little one(s)... I truly believe that we can keep on shifting the dynamics here on Earth, one gentle birth at a time... :)

Angela Stokes-Monarch
Vilcabamba, Ecuador,
March 2012

Contents:

Introduction

Our Intentions for The Future

Introduction

I want to make it very clear that I make *no* claim whatsoever to be an "expert" in the field of pregnancy/birthing/parenting… I'm simply excited to share my journey in this arena, along with the information that I found to be the most useful on my way. We gave birth to our first child, our dear little daughter, Oria Berry Monarch, on November the 20th, 2011. Oria joined us via a swift and smooth, unassisted, lotus waterbirth, in our bath at home, in Vilcabamba, Ecuador.

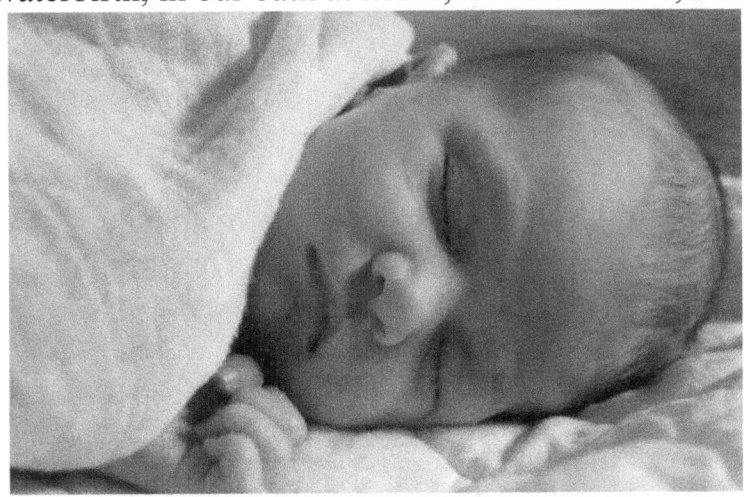

I'm excited to share here everything that I found useful to know for pregnancy, birthing and life immediately post-partum – all of the things that I would have loved to have been told, or to have found in one book, rather than reading dozens and dozens of books to piece together the things that resonated for me…
I suspect that much of what I share here would be more useful for other *new* mums to hear though, rather than more experienced mamas ;)

I also want to make it clear from the start of this book that I intend to discuss here only the *"positive"* choices we have made and continue to make in terms of parenting. There are so many myriad things we have chosen *not* to partake in or do not intend to implement as our child grows up. It is not my desire to go into *why* we choose not to do each of these things, as for me it is clear that none of these things seem like optimal well-being practices and hence we choose alternatives. There are also countless "alternative" parenting books out there outlining over and over again why these things may not be the wisest choices, so…there's plenty already out there to explore on these topics if you want more information…

The kind of things we do *not* choose to engage in include: ultrasounds, internal pregnancy check-ups, medicalised/hospital birth with bright lights/clinical environment/strangers/monitors/time limits/restrictions on eating or drinking, inductions, birthing drugs, epidurals, elective Caesarean sections, extra people at the birth, episiotomies, circumcision, umbilical cord cutting, vaccines, eye drops at birth, separation at birth, bottle feeding formula, nappy (diaper) wearing, setting babies to sleep in another room, cots (cribs), letting babies "cry it out", schedules, using pushchairs (strollers) with very young babies, using dummies (pacifiers), giving allopathic medicines, day care, schooling, non-organic food, non-"eco" clothing/toys and so on… I list these here simply to give you an idea of the kind of things I'm *not* excited to discuss in this book – so from here on out we'll leave these practices and discussions to others…

I feel that it is so important for pregnant women to focus on *positive* birth stories and information, as there seems to be such a culture of *fear* around childbirth and parenting in our current societies. Do your best to be connected to positive, uplifting stories, whether through reading, watching videos online or speaking with other "conscious" parents. If people start to share their fears and "horror stories" around birthing and parenting with you, remember that you do *not* have to listen or dwell on these ideas – they are someone else's story, not something you have to be connected to…keep it positive :) I hope that this book is useful for you in this regard too…

Please also keep in mind that all babies are individuals and have their own paths to unfold. Please do not be fearful if you read anything here that doesn't match with your experiences – I am just sharing one story and one perspective. If you and I both had new puppies in our homes, we wouldn't expect their lives, patterns, development and personalities to be exact replicas of each other – it's just the same with babies; they're all different.

Please note that I've done my best throughout this ebook to *hyperlink* all book names, DVD titles, supplements, clothing items and other products, so that you can easily locate these items for sale online. Just hover your mouse over any product name in this ebook and all being well you ought to be able to just click right there on that name to open a new internet window and see the product online.

Lastly, please understand that I am British and use British spelling/grammar/words, so if you see an "s" where you might expect a "z", an extra "u" here and there that you're not used to, or mention of "nappies" rather than "diapers", it's just the UK way, not a faulty spell checker… ;)

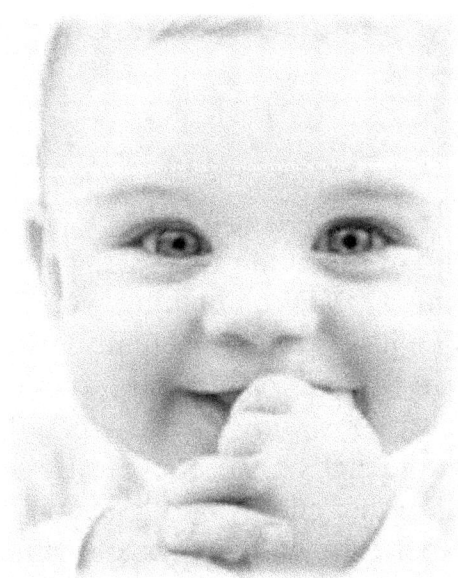

Pregnancy

Conscious Conception

Mr. Monarch and I did a *lot* of preparation prior to conceiving Oria – we were literally reading books, watching DVDs and taking workshops on conscious parenting for *years* prior to it feeling like it was time to actually bring someone in… People often seemed to think we were strange for focusing so much on this subject when we weren't even pregnant and I was*constantly* asked by people if I was in fact pregnant – it seemed strange to most people that we were preparing so much in advance.
However, we chose to put all of that energy and focus on this subject because we both felt like we had almost no experience with babies and children and we knew we didn't want to follow the "mainstream" model of child-rearing, so we were doing our best to research what we might love to do instead.

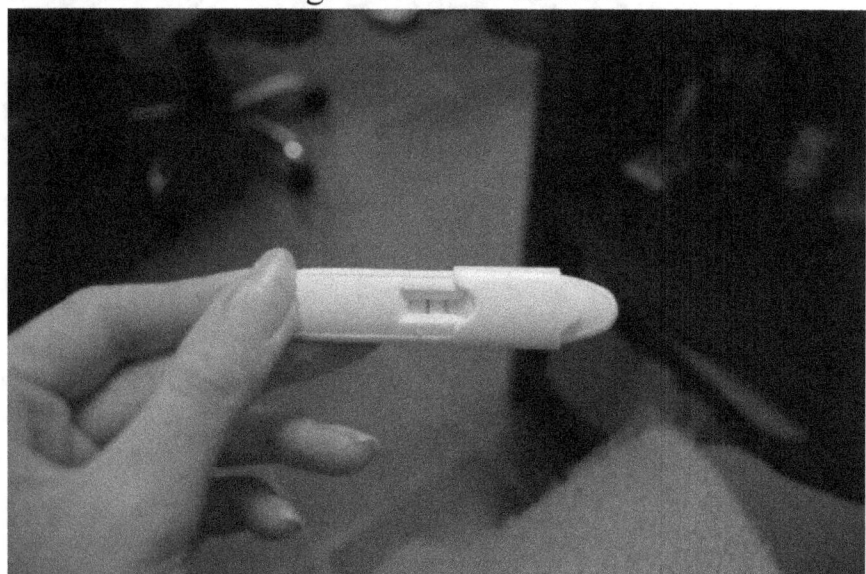

One thing that became clear for us was that we wanted to *consciously* conceive our child, i.e. to express our preferences for a child to the Universe and consciously welcome in whoever might want to join us here. This we did and on the third month of trying, we were blessed to conceive Oria. Apparently it takes an average of five months usually, for couples to conceive. The night I did a pregnancy urine test and saw those two little lines for the first time, showing that we were indeed pregnant, we were in bliss and my life was forever changed. From the moment we saw those two lines, my whole being became focused on the new life that was apparently coming to join us…my thoughts were filled with all things baby and parent and we were so excited for the unfolding journey :)

Nausea/Morning Sickness

I didn't ever vomit during pregnancy, however I did experience quite a lot of nausea, mainly in weeks 3-8. The best way I found to deal with the nausea was to not focus on it – I found that focusing on things outside of myself, especially in terms of being kind to others, helped me to allow the nausea to pass. I was acutely aware during this nausea period that every bite of food required "negotiation" to get it past my lips. I felt compelled to warn my stomach in advance of every bite I intended to consume and wait for feedback on whether this would be acceptable or not. I also couldn't really bare to hear people talk about or even mention foods – my stomach would turn for example at even the mention of something such as "almond butter", which I would usually love and relish.

After weeks 3-8 I didn't seem to deal so much with nausea as experience indigestion issues when eating. At pretty much every meal, I'd feel the strong urge to get up and walk around during eating, to release built-up air bubbles in my stomach. Then I'd feel able to sit down and eat more.

It seems to me that women often feel impelled to only eat simple foods once they are pregnant. So, to make the process easier on ourselves, it might be wise for women to start eating more simply in the six months or so *prior to conception*, if possible. This will mean less detox to experience if you do feel compelled to eat very simply once pregnant, hence less nausea/ill-feeling – nice ;) "Eating more simply" will of course look different for each person, depending on the background they are coming from…this might include reducing/eliminating things like processed starches, refined sugars, excito-toxins, "junk" food, trans-fats, artificial sweeteners, factory-farmed animal products, caffeine and so on…you are the best judge of what might make sense for *you* as a step closer to simplicity.

Cravings/Eating

I did not experience any particular or unusual food cravings during pregnancy. People had warned me a lot in advance that I may not be able to continue to eat totally raw "bee-gan" *(i.e. raw vegan with some bee products)*, might crave foods from my youth and so on – none of this turned out to be true for me though… I continued to eat pretty much exactly as I had before, just a more limited range of things, as my body was reluctant to accept some things. Like many other women, green juice became very challenging for me to ingest earlier in the pregnancy, though I was fine again with it in later months… The best explanation I've heard for this issue with greens was via our dear raw friend and author Shazzie, who told me that the greens are "rejected" because the baby's liver is not yet developed well enough to handle them…hmmmmmmm, makes sense to me…

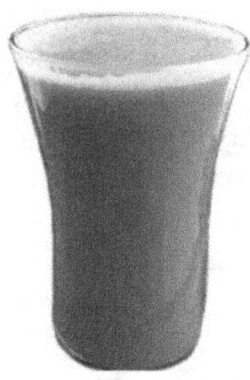

Eating very often felt like hard work to me during pregnancy, requiring concentration, negotiation, attention; it was definitely not something very pleasurable and felt more like a "chore", which is pretty odd to experience for someone coming from a background of overeating on a massive scale.

Here are a few examples of what a typical day's intake for me during pregnancy as a 100% raw "bee-gan" usually looked like – these food logs are all taken straight from my blog (rawreform.blogspot.com), where I have recorded my intake daily since 2006:

1 quart water
1 cup mandarin/orange juice
1 quart greeeeeen juice mixed with pineapple juice
little bowl of strawberries with mango
bowl of yummmmmers fresh salad from the garden mixed with avocado, coconut vinegar, chlorella flakes and lecithin, followed by a couple of dried persimmons with Pili Nut butter
water of two young coconuts

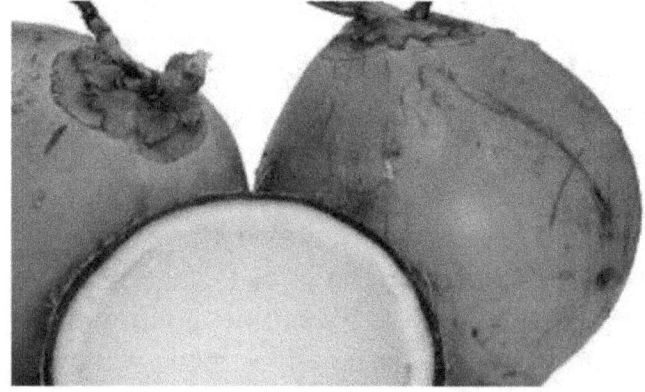

or:

1 quart water

1 cup mandarin/orange/passionfruit juice
2 cups coconut water blended with Elixir of The Lake
chunk of fresh, amazing cherimoya
bowl of energy soup from the garden with avo, sauerkraut, nori on the side, followed
by a little hand-made raw carob confectionary :)
water of two young coconuts
a few yummmmers fresh strawberries and blackberries
2 cups water

or:

1 quart water
1 cup coconut water/orange juice
30 chlorella tablets
little bowl of fresh fruit (granadilla, papaya), with Lydia's Berry Cereal and coconut
water
2 cups coconut water
little bowl of cucumber salad with Mr. M; salad stuffed into handmade flax wraps
with Sea Clear, tahini and sauerkraut, followed by some dried Jackfruit
2 cups water
2 cups coconut water
a sliced apple with molten white Pili Nut "Chocolate"

If some of the terms in these food logs are unfamiliar to you, such as Pili Nut
"Chocolate", chlorella tablets, Elixir of The Lake, coconut vinegar and so on, you can
find all of these kind of products and much more in our online
store, www.TheRawFoodWorld.com - the biggest online raw food and superfood
store in the world.

Raw, Organic, Wild

I suspect that for most of you reading this, there's no need for me to explain the fact
that our family chooses to eat raw vegan/bee-gan and organic or wild-crafted foods.
However, in the interest of those who may not be familiar with these ideas, I'll briefly
explain our perspective.

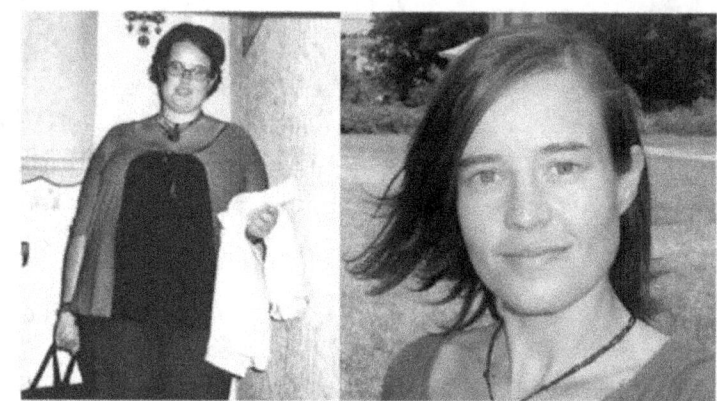

My husband has been eating totally raw vegan/bee-gan for around 15 years as I write this and I've been on this path for about 10 years, since 2002. I used to weigh almost 300lbs before choosing a raw lifestyle – going raw helped me release around 160lbs of excess weight and my life is now basically unrecognisable from before. You can see my before/after pictures and much more on my site: RawReform.com.

We eat raw because we feel that it is the most natural way for humans to eat food, just like all other animals in the wild eat raw, whether they are herbivores, carnivores or omnivores, no-one else cooks their food and we don't either.

Many people report remarkable shifts in their lives from choosing a raw lifestyle, such as more energy, weight loss, diseases reversed, detox, aging reversal, clearer thinking, feeling more connected spiritually and so on. We have a great deal of articles, videos, free e-books and more all about the raw lifestyle that can be accessed at our main site TheRawFoodWorld.com.

As for choosing organic/biodynamic or wild foods, the reasons are myriad: healthier for us and the environment, not contributing to extra pollution, more nutrient density, better taste, stronger connection to nature, no GMOs and so on. There are countless resources these days to explain/support healthier food choices – happy foraging :)

Miscarriage Prevention Brew

At about nine weeks of pregnancy, I had a dream one night that I miscarried. I became concerned that this could be a "premonition", especially when I heard from a friend that miscarriages tend to happen at around twelve weeks of gestation, as there is typically a large hormonal shift around that time. *(Apparently around 1 in 5 human pregnancies usually end in miscarriage – it is very common).*

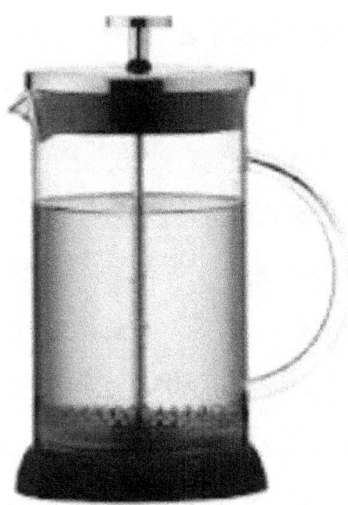

I decided to set my intentions clearly on NOT miscarrying this child and as a back-up, I prepared in a tea-press a mixture of dried herbs mentioned in the fabulous book "Wise Woman Herbal for the Childbearing Year", by Susun Weed. I kept these dry herbs ready in the tea press, near the kettle, in case of any "emergency" situation. I let Mr. M know where this mixture was and that if I ever asked him to go and prepare this tea, to please do so immediately. Fortunately I never felt the need to have this tea prepared. It felt very reassuring for me though, to know that this powerful brew was waiting there to help us *if* we required it. The recommended mixture is: 1oz wild yam, 1oz squaw vine (also known as partridgeberry), ½ oz cramp bark. Simmer herbs with 1 quart water for 20 minutes and then drink a few ounces every four hours until miscarriage symptoms stop.

Check-Ups

The only health check-ups I had during pregnancy were with an 82-year-old man named Polivio, starting in week 34 of gestation.

I was concerned that the baby was in an other-than-optimal position for birthing and a friend suggested we go to see Polivio, who has been helping out women in our area here in Ecuador with their pregnancies and births for *decades* and specialises in turning babies who are in awkward positions. So off we went for our $5 appointment with Don Polivio…and indeed it turned out that Oria *was* in an unusual position…she was set up at that point to come out *feet*-first, as a "footling breech" – eeeeeeeek… Polivio got to work and turned her from the outside, using nothing but his hands and decades of experience. Turning a baby from the outside like this is known as "external version" by midwives and is not a very common skill these days, it seems. It was quite painful for me to experience this turning, yet the pain lasted only a few short minutes, then it was done – far preferable to potential *hours* of challenge trying to birth a breech baby, in my opinion. I felt soooooo extremely grateful to Polivio for moving Oria into an optimal position for us. I saw him two times more before birthing, just so he could check that she'd remained in situ. Indeed she had and was born easily in 1 hour 17 minutes, head-first, in the optimal position – hurray :)

There are many other natural ways to turn breech babies too, if you don't have someone around you who can perform "external version" – you can use slant boards, spend time on all-fours daily, do visualisations, spend time in water, use homeopathic remedies and so on.

Rest/Stress/Sleep

I believe that it's vital for pregnant women to get plenty of rest and be as stress-free as possible, for an optimal gestation to unfold. I was given repeated messages from my body to *slow down* during pregnancy. I thought I already was living a pretty slow life, yet the messages kept on coming to slow down even more, so I did… Lots of reading, lots of laying down, deep breathing, meditation, gentle stretching, massages. I did my very best to stay focused on positive things during my pregnancy too, despite the fact that some very challenging things were unfolding for us at that time…I chose to spiral *upwards* as best I could and to only engage in the absolute minimum possible of details about anything that felt challenging. Remember, the baby feels *everything* that you feel.

For most of the pregnancy, I slept well. Things became more challenging in the latter months however, as I have always slept on my front and from about month five/six, my belly was getting too big to lay on my front anymore… Learning to sleep on my side instead felt really uncomfortable and strange at first. At the same time, I was starting to become a little bit of an insomniac as well in the last trimester, which felt really odd too. I began to kind of dread going to bed. I later realised I was most likely experiencing a massive need for *calcium* at that point, as I was craving tahini like crazy (very rich in calcium), insomnia is related to calcium needs and the baby was in a big phase of growing right then… For anyone else in this situation, I'd suggest taking Calcium Angstrom Mineral, drinking Natural Calm, eating calcium-rich foods like leafy greens, tahini and dried apricots and even taking products like "Bone Response" or "Bone Renewal". I also found a few drops of Skullcap Tincture to be invaluable for helping me to get to sleep.

Chiming

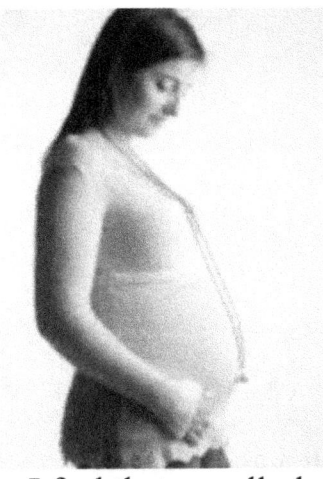

I feel that a really lovely gift for pregnant women is a "Chime" necklace, also sometimes known as a Mexican "Bola Harmony" ball necklace. These necklaces usually involve a very long chain, reaching all the way down to the growing belly, with a little ball pendant attached, which chimes as the woman moves around. Apparently from around 20 weeks of age, the fetus can pick up the sounds from outside, so will hear the gentle chiming sound from next to the mum's belly. When the baby is later born, they will associate hearing that gentle chiming sound with being in the comforting embrace of the womb and it can help soothe them.

Supplements

I took a number of supplements during pregnancy and continue to take them all now too, as a breastfeeding mama. I am extremely grateful to our dear friend Shazzie for all of her wonderful research and information on nutrition for pregnancy/breastfeeding, laid out in her fabulous book "Evie's Kitchen". Based on Shazzie's guidance and my own intuition, these are the main "supplements" I've been enjoying *(though the term "supplement" might be a little odd in regards to some of these items, depending on your perspective…)*

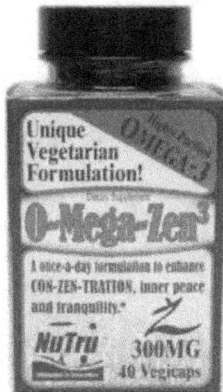

*"Baby and Me" pre-natal whole food tablets from Megafood
*Omega-Zen-3 (for DHA)

*Vitamin B12 patches
*Vitamin K2 caps
*Vitamin D spray
*Non-GMO lecithin powder (for choline, for brain development)
*Andreas' oils
*Bone Response/Bone Renewal
*Natural Calm
*Angstrom minerals of Zinc, Calcium, Iron
*Kelp capsules

I also ate and continue to eat plenty of algaes, like chlorella, spirulina and marine phytoplankton, for their protein and chlorophyll-packed nutrient density.

I did not necessarily remember or *want* to use all of these every day during pregnancy – I took things as often as I remembered and wanted to take them that day. The same pattern applies now as I breastfeed – most days I remember to use most things, however it's not all like clockwork and still all seems to be well…

I chose to use this list of things as I value very much the research and concerns that Shazzie shared about possible deficiencies among vegan/raw children and how best to side-step such deficiencies. I did not want to take any "risks" with our child, so I did the best I could to join the dots. I would strongly encourage others interested in this area to read Shazzie's book and consider carefully their supplementing choices too.

Please also note that it is usually strongly recommended to NOT take any enzyme supplements during pregnancy, especially systemic enzymes, as apparently the enzymes can identify the fetus as "foreign" to the body and go to work dissolving it. I took no enzymes at all during pregnancy, whereas I usually took our potent Systemic Enzyme blend most days prior to pregnancy.

Things to Avoid During Pregnancy

Here below is a list that I compiled a while back of various foods, herbs and activities it is generally recommended to avoid during pregnancy. Please note, these suggestions were sent in by *various* people in response to a question from one of my blog readers. You may not perhaps agree with ALL that is included here, please remember to take in this list with a gentle, open heart and to use your own intuition to guide you as to which of these things may or may not be appropriate for yourself, if you are pregnant or open to new life joining you…

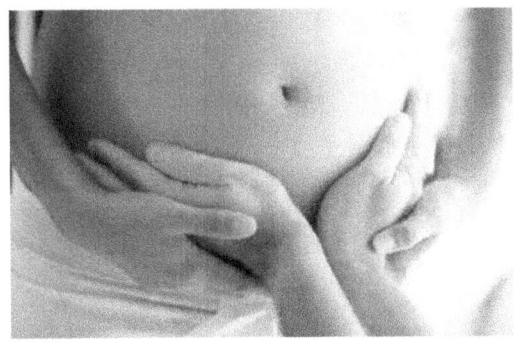

Please note too that there seem to be a lot of issues for pregnant women around meats, shellfish, fish, cheeses and other such items that people sometimes eat - these items are not mentioned in the list below, as this list is primarily focused on raw vegan items...please feel free to research further online if you are concerned about animal products...

Also, alcohol/cigarettes/drugs/caffeine and processed foods are similarly all items not included in the lists below that are clearly best not consumed during pregnancy (*or at **all**, from my perspective...* ;).

There are three sections below of items/activities to be cautious of during pregnancy: foods, herbs and activities; though some of the foods and herbs may overlap each other, I've done my best to divide them up in a way that I think most people can easily relate to:

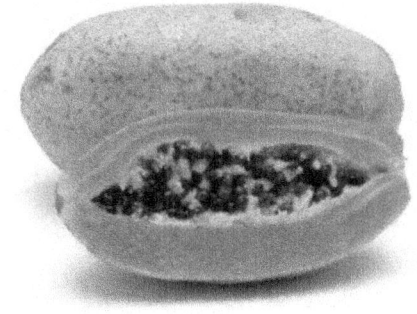

Foods:
Parsley
Cilantro
Garlic
Cayenne/hot spices
Pineapple/papaya (esp seeds)
Sesame seeds
Cacao
Agave

Flax seed
Aloe
Fresh wood sorrel

Herbs:

angelica	ginger	osha root
artemisia	ginseng	passion flower
bethroot	golden seal root	pau d'arco
birthwort	goldenseal	pennyroyal
black cohosh	hops	Peruvian bark
black cohosh	horsetail	rosemary plant in flower
blue cohosh	hyssop leaves	rue leaves
buchu	juniper berries	saffron stigmas
buckthorn	lemon balm	sage
cascara sagrada	licorice	saw palmetto
castor oil	liferoot in flower	senna
cotton root bark	lovage root	sumac berries
ephedra	marijuana female flowers	sweet flag root
ergot fungus	misteltoe leaves	tansy leaves
European vervain plant	motherwort	turkey rhubarb
feverfew plant in flower	mugwort	yohimbe

*Much of the above list was compiled from the fabulous book "Wise Woman Herbal for The Childbearing Year" by Susun Weed.

*Master Herbalist Susun Weed also has a little article HERE on herbs that are *supportive* during pregnancy.

*There is also a big list of suggested herbs to avoid here:
http://www.herb-health-guide.com/herbs-to-avoid-during-pregnancy.html
(*note, some of the "culinary" herbs are said to be ok in food prep in small amounts, not in "medicinal" doses though…e.g. basil, caraway seeds, celery seed, fresh horseradish, savory, majoram, nutmeg, rosemary, saffron, tarragon, thyme, watercress…*)

Activities/States:

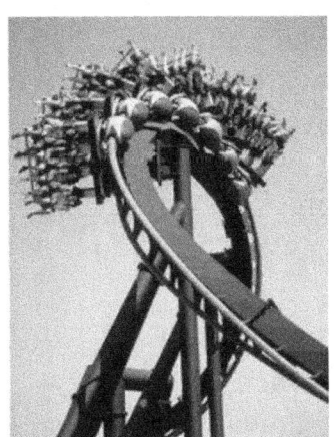

*Stress
*Contact with cat litter and other animal feces
*Contact with pesticides/pollutants/toxins/paint fumes/household chemicals/hair dyes and so on
*Fasting
*Electric blankets and water beds
*Ultrasounds and x-rays
*Amusement park rides
*Taking systemic enzymes, ascorbic acid, antihistamines, antacids, laxatives, diuretics
*Tight clothing, high heeled shoes
*Standing for extended periods of time
*Loud noises (e.g. concerts)
*Airplane travel, any lengthy travel

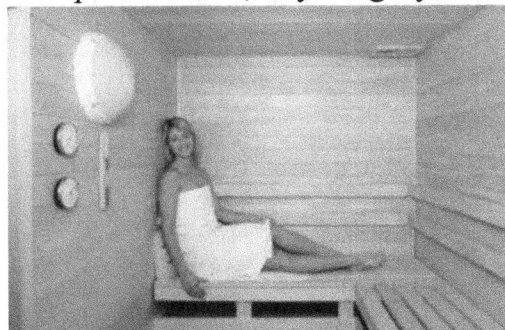

*Hot baths/saunas/hot tubs/hot yoga/any activity or situation where you could become very hot
*Strenuous/vigorous activities, especially in the third trimester e.g. kickboxing, intense hiking, scuba diving, trampolining, weight lifting, horseriding - any activities where there is the chance to fall, where balance is key or where high altitudes are involved
*Some yoga poses that put pressure on the belly, plus any exercises such as abdominal crunches that exert pressure on the abdominal muscles

I really hope that this list helps add some value and support to your journey. Remember to use your own intuition as to which foods and so on are appropriate to you - and if you are pregnant and have been consuming/doing anything on this list, I would strongly encourage you *not* to go into any feelings of fear or "self-blame", remember that these are all just *suggestions*, from various sources - *you* are your own best guide for what feels appropriate to you. Huge thanks to everyone who contributed to this list of suggestions.

External Influences

I would encourage being very cautious during pregnancy about which kinds of external influences you allow into your life, in the form of media, music, conversations, social contexts and so on. Remember: your baby feels everything that you feel and has no filter to determine, for example, if you are feeling "fear" because there is a genuine physical threat in your vicinity or because you're watching a scary film. Do your best to maintain a calm, loving, uplifting emotional environment for your baby to thrive in, rather than exposing yourself and therefore them too, to depressing, upsetting or disturbing experiences.

A Private Pregnancy

We chose not to tell anyone about our pregnancy until Oria had safely arrived Earthside. We didn't even tell our families or the people who live with us here on our land. The main reason for this was that we were making some rather "unconventional" choices around pregnancy/birthing/child-raising and we did not want to have other peoples' fears, criticisms and projections pointed at us before Oria even arrived here. We wanted the energetic field around her gestation and birth to be as "clean", positive and supported as possible. One of the unfortunate realities of living life "in public" as Mr. M and I currently do, through our videos, newsletters, talks, blogs and so on, is that there seems to always be a certain number of people who do not appreciate the work we are sharing and are very vocal in expressing their criticisms and "negativity" towards us. We did not want Oria to be subjected to this kind of energy in the womb, so we kept our pregnancy entirely secret to help protect her.

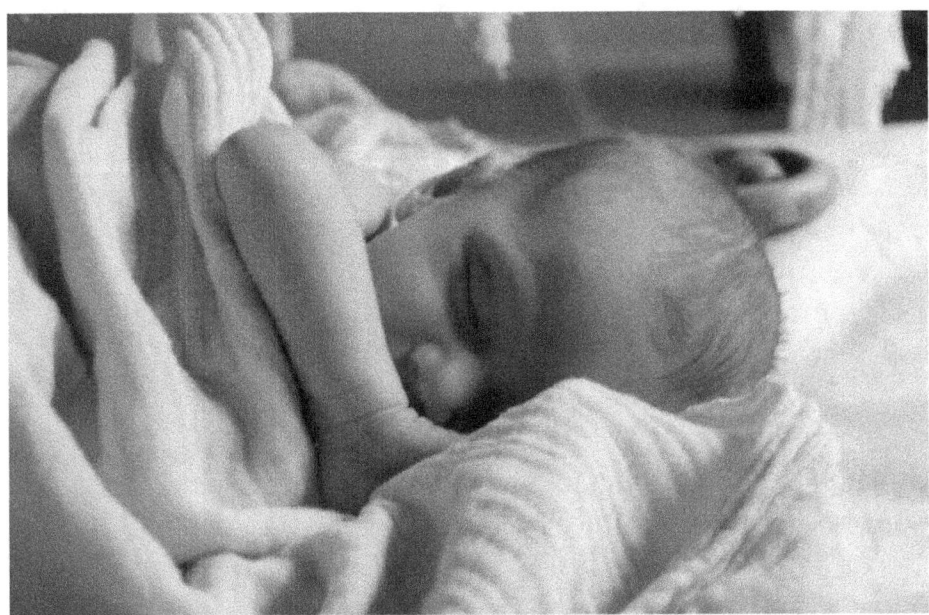

It all worked out well in the end, though it did start to feel pretty silly for me personally in the final couple of months of pregnancy as I repeatedly told well-meaning local friends "no, I'm not pregnant", when I clearly had a huge belly bundled up beneath my baggy clothes ;) Usually people would just conclude I'd regained some extra weight and drop the subject. Being social at that time did feel quite awkward to me though, so I kept things pretty low-key socially for those last couple of months... I was also feeling very emotionally sensitive, vulnerable and easily moved to tears during pregnancy, so it felt easier for me to not be around many people for this reason too.

Strange Bodily Changes

Women's bodies of course go through enormous changes during pregnancy and many shifts are easy to anticipate, such as expanding belly and breasts, possible nausea, stretch marks and so on. However, there were quite a few bodily changes I experienced during pregnancy that I hadn't been so much anticipating...

For example, I had quite a few **nosebleeds** during pregnancy, which is actually a common issue, related to the increase in blood volume as the body works to produce another being. For me the nosebleeds started around the end of the third month/start of the fourth and continued occasionally through the fifth and sixth months too. I would mostly experience them at night or first thing in the morning; the bleeding would start suddenly, last a few minutes with fairly heavy, bright red blood-flow, then stop. It was more of an inconvenience than any great concern...

Another strange bodily reaction to get used to was sudden **sharp, driving pains** in the chest as my breasts were changing and expanding, in preparation for lactation. Again, this was of no great concern, just a natural consequence of the huge bodily changes underway.

Later in pregnancy, it began to feel increasingly **challenging to sit down**, as it felt like things in my abdomen would "compress" (unsurprisingly of course, given that another entire human being was occupying my womb ;). There just wasn't as much room in that area of my body anymore and it felt like everything "squished" together as I'd sit down, creating discomfort for a few seconds. Travelling in vehicles on bumpy roads began to feel very uncomfortable too, as my abdomen felt stuffed and vulnerable to the jostling motions.

It was also increasingly challenging to touch my toes by six months and onwards…this reminded me a lot of being in a morbidly obese body…socks were tough to get on and slip-on shoes were definitely favoured.

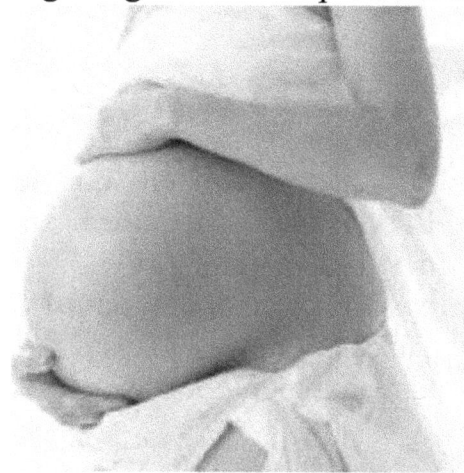

Though I lived in a morbidly obese body for many years and know what it feels like to be heavy, being pregnant was different…I actually felt more "debilitated" as a heavily *pregnant* woman, as there were various activities I didn't feel safe/confident to undertake now (e.g. bike-riding, trampolining, flying in planes), whereas as a heavily obese person, I'd rarely let anything get in my way and was typically very active.

I also noticed that in the later months of pregnancy it often felt challenging for me to **urinate**. It felt like things were not set up in the same way anymore in my abdomen and it was now necessary to *concentrate*, to be able to get the urine out… I also seemed to be urinating more frequently in those latter months, as there was less space for the bladder to fill out, so it required emptying more often.

Another unusual bodily experience I had during pregnancy was **partial hearing loss**. I have fairly low blood pressure and would find at times that it seemed my body was so busy working in my abdomen that it didn't have enough spare resources to pump blood efficiently all the way up to my head to keep my hearing functioning optimally. Again, this was more of an inconvenience than anything else and I was happy that my body, in its infinite wisdom, was prioritising the baby's development over anything else. I could always get my hearing back fully whenever I wanted, by laying down and especially by elevating my legs while laying down.

I became extremely *slooooooooooooow* physically in the first trimester of pregnancy especially. I started to notice for example that my morning yoga/movement/meditation practice, which would usually take me thirty minutes or so, was now taking at least twice as long. I was fine with this shift and happy to take things more slowly, however I can imagine that some women would find this change in pace challenging to adapt to.

I noticed an increased amount of **spots** (pimples) on my shoulders and upper back during pregnancy. I am not entirely sure what this indicated, though I imagine my liver was struggling to keep up with all the extra waste to manage…

While I definitely anticipated feeling the baby kicking and moving around inside me, the reality of actually experiencing this in my body was quite something… It often felt like **motion sickness** to me when the baby was moving around, as the movements felt so dramatic and were not coming from "me" – I was being moved by something else… I would mostly feel the baby moving at night when I would first get into bed and lay on my back and then also when I would first sit at my desk in the morning – I guess she didn't like the sudden "compressed" feeling of me sitting down after a night of more spacious expansion ;) Apparently many babies like to move around most at night, as their mums are most relaxed then, so there's more space to shift in the womb…and this can lead to babies being rather wakeful at night for the first few days or weeks after they arrive Earthside…

Affirmations and Fear-Busting

I'd love to share here about a couple of written exercises I did during pregnancy that I really enjoyed. The first was simply writing a list of positive affirmations for myself around the theme of pregnancy, birthing and parenting, for example:

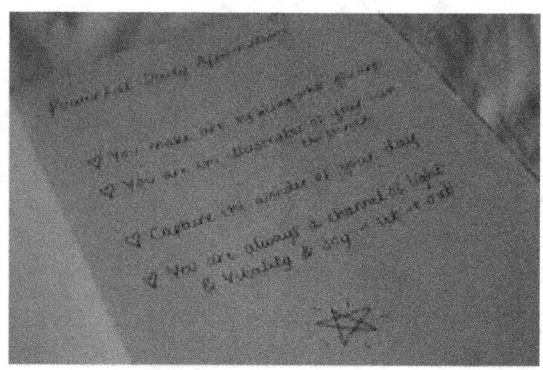

This baby is healthy.
This baby feels loved.
This baby knows we are excited to meet them.
This baby is going to be in the optimal position for birth.
This baby is going to be born gently and swiftly into water.
We are going to birth unassisted, easily and safely.
This baby will feel welcomed and secure from birth.
We will enjoy a peaceful, loving and rich baby moon together.
My body is going to heal rapidly and well after birth.
This baby will grow up surrounded with love, affection and compassion.

I always make sure to use *positive* wording with affirmations, e.g. stating what I *am* excited for, rather than using phrases such as "I don't/can't/won't…" and so on. I would look at this list from time to time to remind myself of what I wanted to co-create.

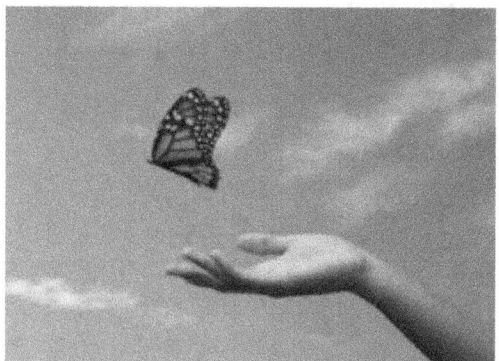

Another exercise that I found really rewarding was something suggested in the "Birthing From Within" book by Pam England and Rob Horowitz. Firstly I wrote out all of the myriad fears that I could possibly find in my head about pregnancy/birthing/parenting, then on another page I drew some images to represent the *optimal* outcomes I could perceive around these areas, e.g. ecstatic birth despite whatever circumstances may arise, feelings of love, empowerment, clarity, support and so on. This exercise felt extremely "cleansing" for me. I actually read out my page of fears to Mr. M after I was done with this exercise and we just *laughed* at them, as by then the energy had been transformed and my concerns seemed rather silly – what a wonderful way to bust through those fears, giving voice to them so that they can be dissolved and instead creating positive imagery to focus on and enjoy… :)

Communication

I believe that it is very wise for potential parents-to-be to discuss various ideas around pregnancy/birthing/parenting before even *conceiving*, if possible, or at least prior to the baby's birth, to see how you can successfully align your thoughts and visions together. According to the "Birthing From Within" book, only one in five marriages is reported to "improve" after the birth of a child; most go into "decline" and the spouses reportedly argue a lot more than before. Soooooo, with that in mind, you might want to consider getting very clear *before*-hand on things such as: birthing choices, food choices, education, vaccination, involvement of other family members with your child, what to do if the child injures themselves, what to do if the child takes something from another child, communication concerns, values you would/wouldn't like to pass on to the child and so on. Getting clear on all of these kinds of topics and more, *before* you're immersed in full-on childcare can help things to flow much more smoothly…

…and on the subject of communicating with your partner, or any other caretakers of your child: once the child is here, try not to turn your conversation into a "competition" of who is the most tired/stressed/hard-working and so on…instead do your best to be supportive of each other and to focus on and celebrate the *great* things that are happening: you got three hours sleep in a row, the baby smiled today, you were able to get some project done that you're excited about and so on – do your best to keep things positive and uplifting… :)

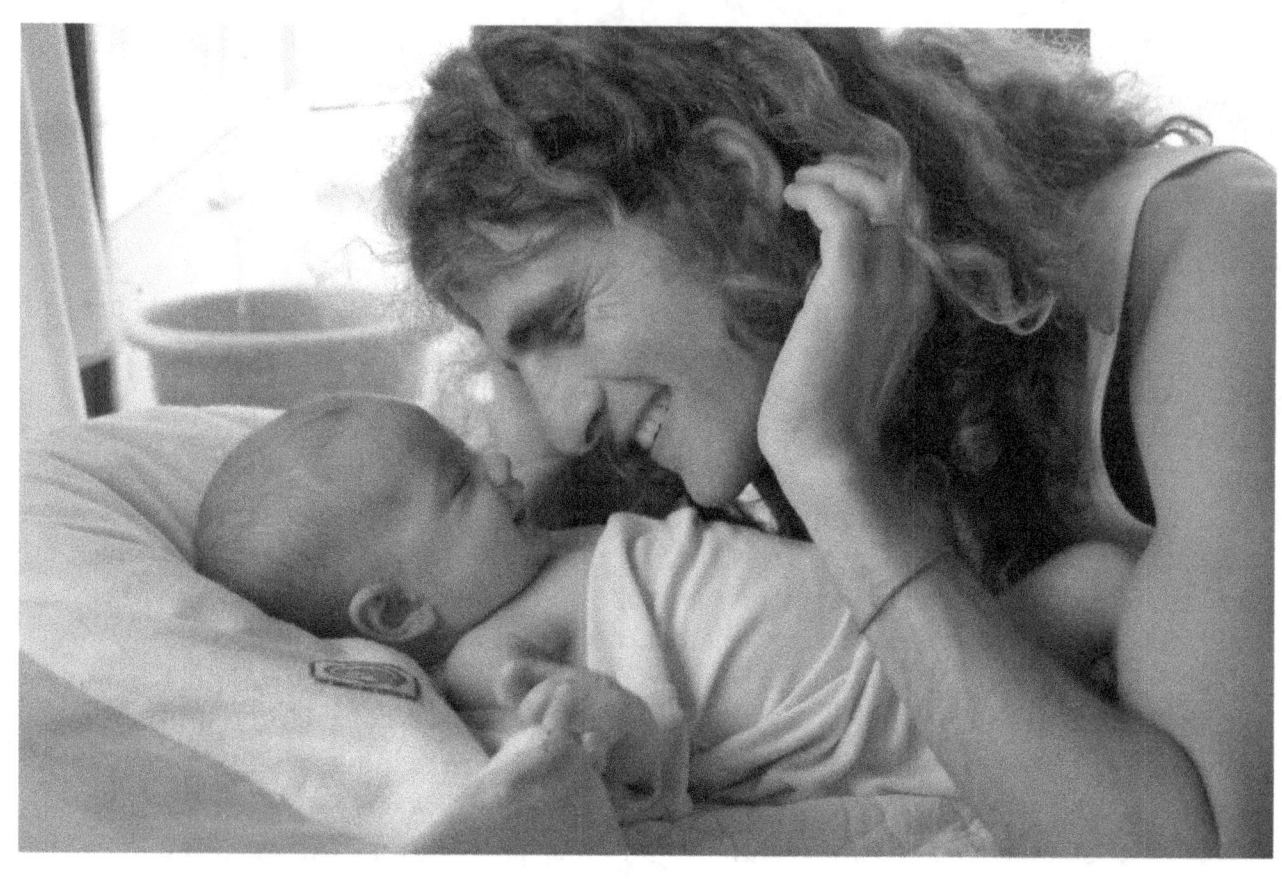

Birth

The Birth of Oria Berry Monarch

I anticipated the arrival of our baby around December the 9th, 2011, as that seemed to me to be around the time we'd hit 40 weeks and there was a full moon the same week. Well, it turned out Oria had different ideas…

On the morning of November the 20th, I noticed pink spotting on the toilet paper after I urinated…"that's odd" I thought…and went on with the day…I was feeling a little strange in the abdomen, with mild sensations similar to menstrual cramping. After a few hours I decided to tell Mr. M that something felt different – I wasn't sure what was going on – I just wanted him to be in on whatever was unfolding…then after a while it crossed my mind that maybe this was the start of *labour*… I didn't want to give energy to that thought though, as in my ideal picture, we were still about 2.5 weeks away from birth. I kept suggesting to the baby to NOT come now, if that was indeed what was starting to unfold…well, again, Oria had different ideas ;)

I went on with the day with strange abdominal sensations, yet still not *really* knowing that I was in labour… then at one point in the evening I went to the bathroom and this time the toilet paper was red with blood…oh… Now I knew something was definitely happening. I started to make my way to the front of the house, to try to find Mr. M, who had been outside playing basketball for many hours. Just as I burst through the door to the living room, he entered the room too from outside, exhausted from intense hours on the court. I hurriedly told him that it seemed like I was in labour and we started bustling about, gathering all the various supplies for the bathroom that we wanted to have on hand.

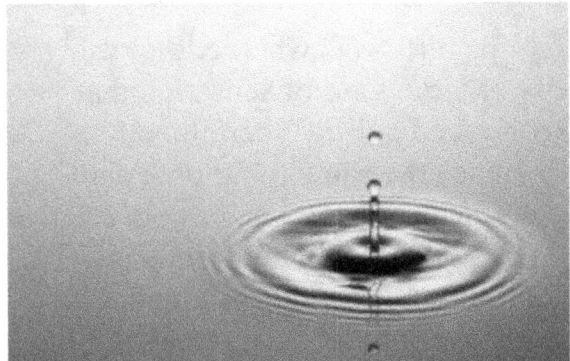

Out in our outside bathroom, I was in the midst of preparing things when suddenly my waters broke with a huge EXPLOSION, all over the floor…it was apparently 7.30pm at that point, Mr. M later told me… He was at the other end of the house right then – I tried shouting to him to let him know what was happening, as liquid gushed out of me seemingly endlessly…after a while he appeared and I was pretty much gone by that point into the right-brain swirl of "labour-land" – I was totally over-awed by the mass of liquid now covering the entire bathroom floor – I couldn't stop staring at it and talking about it – it felt like witnessing something in a film, rather than my actual life – itseemed so very odd, this huge explosion of water all over everything…I was captivated…

Thankfully Mr. M still had his left-brain in operation and was getting all the final things into place for us to get into the bath and bring this baby Earthside.

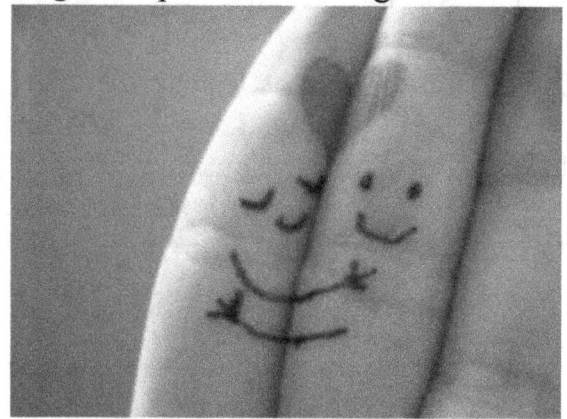

We got into the warm water of our thankfully huge, two-person bath. Mr. M sat beside me on my left, while I positioned myself in an all fours/kind of floating/belly-down position. I was totally gone in labour-land by then, unable to really speak/communicate, all focus and energy directed to working with the contractions/rushes, which were now coming fairly fast and strong. I had two of the fingers of Mr. M's left hand in my left hand and I would squeeeeeeeeeeze them like crazy with every rush. (We were grateful that we had read just that day in one book to not give a labouring woman more than two fingers at a time to squeeze, otherwise she may easily break one or more of the digits from the force of her squeeeeezing – eeeeeeek ;)

One of the things people ask me most often about this birth was whether the rushes were painful. I find this a little challenging to answer…the kind of sensation that comes with each rush is like nothing I'd ever experienced before – certainly not *pleasurable*, in the sense that I'd want to experience the same thing on a daily basis, but not painful in any sense of the word that I suspect would be easy to relate to unless one has given birth. It felt all-consuming…as midwife and author Ina May Gaskin puts it, the rushes required "all of my attention"…I was totally gone in the right-brain, flowing reality of labour-land, not really available to analyse whether I was in pain or not… I will say this though: at the end of it all, it certainly didn't feel to me like something I would *never* choose to do again – it didn't feel overly unmanageable.

With his right hand, Mr. M was applying pressure to my perineum with each contraction/rush, to support the tissue there. Living and breathing through the rushes felt like a huge exercise in focused awareness for me – being with the energy flow, breathing, working out how to flow best with this enormous energy channelling through me. After a few more rushes, my body was in the phase where pushing down was the action being called for – the impulse to push down was all-consuming and clear. I reached down after a while and could feel the baby starting to crown. I could feel a very *peculiar*-feeling shape emerging – I was wondering what it *was* – it didn't feel to me like it could be part of the baby's *head*...I was recalling a friend's birth story of her little boy who arrived testicles-first as a "Frank Breech" and began to wonder if that was what was happening here... I just didn't know...and anyway, it didn't matter...this baby was coming out, head-first or otherwise...

It took me a few contractions more to get my head around how to work most optimally with these rushes...I realised it would work best if I started to push hard *right at the start* of the next rush, so that I'd be able to push enough in the space of one rush to get the head out. I decided to tell Mr. M my realisation. I went to tell him and suddenly found that it was almost impossible for me to speak right then...my voice came out as the faintest, rasping whisper and it felt extremely taxing to get the words out at all, however I wanted him to know what was happening and to be ready for the emergence of the baby. When I told him the baby had been crowning for a while and I was going to try to get the head out on the next rush, he was shocked – he had no idea we were so far along in the process – he thought we were likely going to be there in the bath for many hours more...

Mr. M moved a bit to see better what was happening and as the next rush flowed in, I did my best to work strongly with it... Push, PuSSShhHH, PUUUUUUUUSSSSSSSSSSHHHHHHHHHHHHHH and voila, the head was out. There was Oria's little head, eyes open, looking around and up at her daddy, through the water. Mr. M was ecstatic, while I was focused on getting the body out with the next rush.

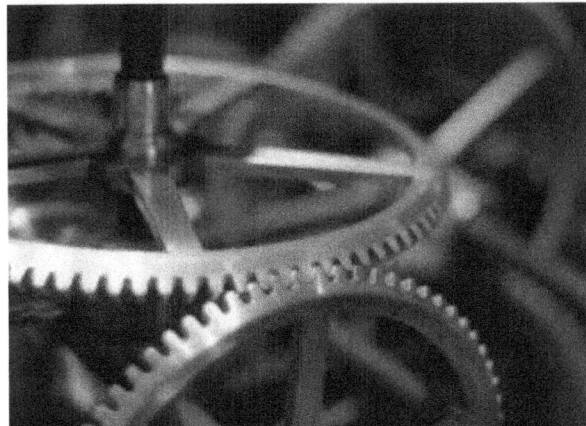

Suddenly the strangest sensations swept through my birthing canal area – on hindsight I imagine this was simply the sensation experienced as Oria's body was turning into the optimal position to then come out on the next rush. At the time however, I was totally baffled by this sensation and kept asking Mr. M what he was *doing* – it felt to me like he was applying pressure with both hands and moving things around – it felt like everything was shifting around like cogs in a clock or something – I *kept* asking Mr. M what he was doing and he kept telling me that he wasn't even touching me at that point, he was just supporting Oria's head – this strange sensation only went on for a number of seconds though before the next rush brought Oria's body sailing out into the water and she was fully here :) It was 8.47pm, an hour and 17 minutes after my water had broken…

I turned around carefully from my "all-fours" position then, lifting my leg over the umbilical cord, to see Mr. M raising our baby up from the water. That moment will be forever etched in my memory, I am sure. I turned and saw this tiny, wriggling human in my husband's hands and…I went into shock… Did that come out of *me*…? I just couldn't get my head around it at first. It looked like a *doll*, but it was moving…it was a real human being…even though I'd obviously known that I was pregnant and that a baby human was the natural consequence of that, nothing had prepared me for that actual moment of coming eye-to-eye, face-to-face with this little person who had just emerged from my body and for whose well-being I was now suddenly responsible…it was all feeling totally surreal to me…

I also couldn't understand at first if this baby was a boy or a girl. I knew that babies' genitals and breast tissue are often swollen at birth from all the mother's hormones, yet I just didn't know what I was looking at – at first I wondered if this was a boy with no penis, which was scary…then we realised that we were apparently just seeing swollen vaginal labia, rather than testicles… We had a girl :) That was our desire and intention from the start and now here she was – so beautiful…

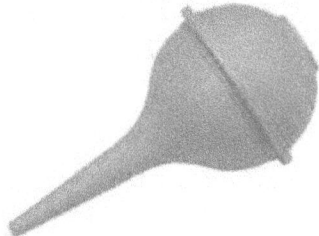

We then used the only piece of equipment that we utilised during the birth, which was a little bulb syringe, to clear mucus out of her mouth and nose… We also had "surgical" scissors and a little plastic umbilical clamp on hand if we had felt the need to cut the umbilical cord, which we didn't – there were no complications and we were able to have the Lotus Birth we desired (see further below).

With Oria's airways clear, we started trying to initiate breastfeeding, however, it wasn't flowing at that point – she wasn't really interested and latching on was actually a challenge for us for the first couple of days. After fifteen minutes or so after her birth, I became concerned that the placenta hadn't yet emerged. I started to focus on that, as I had read that it can be very dangerous for the woman if the placenta is retained. This was actually the most challenging part of the whole birthing process for me, I think – Oria had come out so easily and now the placenta seemed to not be budging and I was getting a little concerned. I tried various things to try to help it to come out – abdominal massage, squatting position, nipple stimulation, trying to get Oria to latch on, pulling the cord gently and so on, however, nothing worked. After a while, we moved to the bed as that is what seemed best to me and Mr. M called our friend Elena Vladirimova, director of the "Birth As We Know It" DVD, to ask her what to do about the placenta. She told him to just pull gently on the umbilical cord, which he came back and did and BAM, there it was suddenly – hurray :) I was sooooo immensely relieved it was out. I took a lot of Shepherd's Purse tincture to help stop the bleeding, which I think really helped, though everything was truly *covered* in blood all around us and I felt very shaky. The bathroom looked like the scene of some horrific atrocity and now the bedroom we were in was splattered with blood in all directions too – bed sheets, floor, towels, clothing, everything…

*(Incidentally, "Unassisted Childbirth" author Laura Shanley later shared with us that she knows people who safely delivered the placenta multiple hours and even**days**after their babies and were fine – Laura encourages women to let the process unfold naturally by itself.)*

With the placenta finally delivered, we all snuggled down into bed to rest. We weighed Oria some hours later when the sun was up again – she was seven and a half pounds, with long, elegant hands, a very healthy, rosy complexion and quite a lot of vernix to rub into her skin.

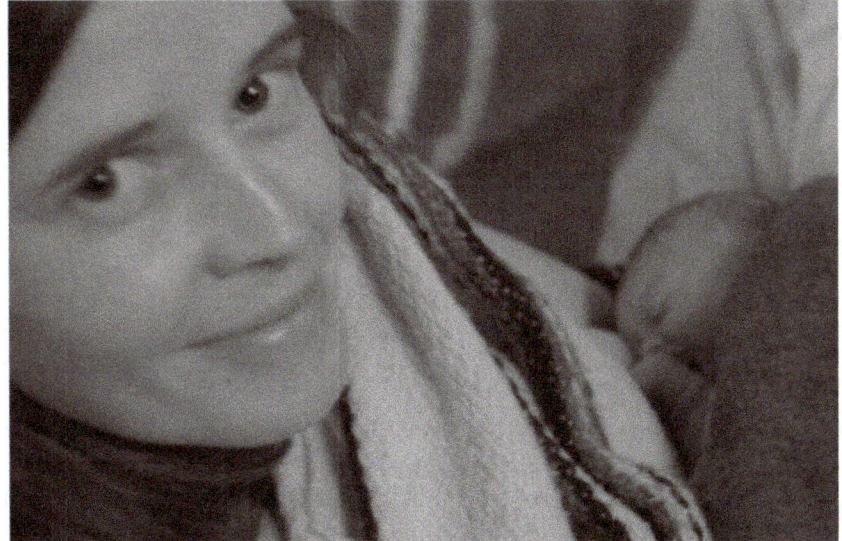

The following hours and days are all a bit of a blur for me – we had entered the newborn-sleep-deprivation-time warp and those first three weeks were all a blur for me of hormone rollercoasters, after-birth contractions and a seemingly endless learning process of how to be with this tiny person, all set to the backdrop of days that turned into nights into days into nights…

Unassisted Birth

Long before Oria was even conceived, we knew that we'd want to have an unassisted childbirth if we were to be blessed with a little one – i.e. just Mr. M and I there to welcome the child, no doctors, midwives, doulas or anyone else. Mammals in the wild almost always choose to birth alone. The presence of other people at a human birth can significantly affect and slow the process.

Not many people seem to realise that we mammals have an inbuilt "fight or flight" response during birthing, in the event that we become upset or startled. For example, as documentary maker Elena Vladirimova explains, if a deer is birthing in the wild and is disturbed by someone or something, her womb will automatically *clamp down*, so that she can get up and run to safety. Now think about this in the context of modern human hospital births, for example, where the birthing woman might be surrounded by many people she doesn't know, bright lights, surgical instruments, IVs, monitors, people barking orders at her and so on…no wonder hospital births tend to have such unfavourable outcomes for people…remember, *we are mammals too…*

One of my personal best role models for birthing was actually our beautiful horse, Barbie *(note: we did**not**choose her name, she came with it ;)*. In the time Barbie has been with us, she has easily and successfully birthed two foals, all by herself, out in the fields around our house. Barbie didn't require a vet, a doctor, bright lights, epidurals or anything else to give birth quickly and easily. In fact, the presence of any of these things would surely have *complicated* and lengthened the process for her. Barbie was my biggest inspiration when considering how I wanted to give birth too and we actually ended up delivering within nine days of each other – Sally Joy, Barbie's little filly, came in on 11-11-11 and Oria Berry joined us nine days later, on 11-20-2011. Both were delivered quickly, smoothly, safely and without the interventions of any external influences. We are so blessed :)

The Cost of Childbirth

The average financial cost of a hospital birth in the USA at present is apparently somewhere around $16,000. This is completely shocking to me. Do animals in the wild *pay* anything to give birth…? Nope… We bought three main things for our birthing process: a bulb syringe, surgical scissors and a plastic umbilical cord clamp; total cost, $12… I know which option makes more sense to me ;)

Similarly, I often hear people commenting on how "expensive" it is to raise children…while I can certainly see how you *could* make it expensive for yourself, with medical fees, schooling fees, masses of clothing, countless toys and children's activities and so on, I definitely don't see it as *inevitable* that having a child must entail huge financial outlays – I believe that it's all a matter of how you choose to raise them…

Awe

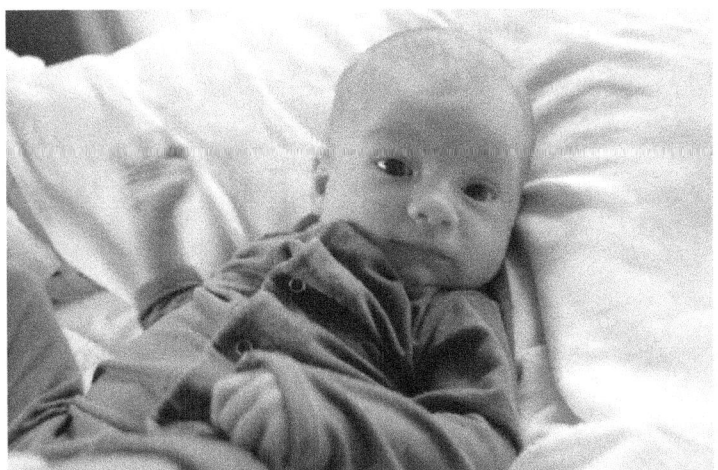

I recall being totally in awe of Oria's existence in her first days here. I just couldn't totally get my head around the fact that my body had apparently created this whole other being… I would look at her hands, the veins under her skin, the tiny fluffy little hairs on her head and I just couldn't quite believe it all…everything was in place, she was totally healthy and complete – how did my body *do* this…? It was so remarkable to me to personally witness that my body has the internal wisdom to be able to create another tiny human. It seemed like this creation had so little to do with any part of me that I might tend to think of as "me" – I wasn't *consciously* working for nine months to make sure all of her organs were developed properly, for example, or that each eyelash was in place and yet, here she was…totally healthy, everything in place…and I was in total awe… :)

Colon Cleansing

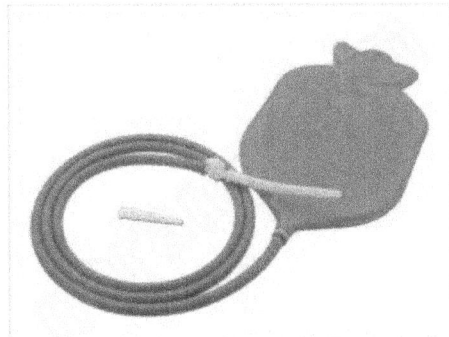

Any of you who are familiar with the work of Mr. M and I will know that we're big proponents of colon cleansing to help people reach and maintain optimal health. Colon cleansing immediately prior to giving birth is a *great* idea, in my opinion, as otherwise women very often release bowel movements during birthing, as they're pushing so hard. In a water birth context this is particularly unfortunate, as it may necessitate the woman getting out of the water. Personally, as I was becoming more and more suspicious that I might be in labour on Oria's birth day, I decided to go and do a colonic that afternoon, using our home unit – and I am so glad I did. Personally I actually did home colonics throughout pregnancy, at least once a week, however, many health care professionals would likely strongly advise women *against* such a practice, through fear… If it feels good to you, you might do colonics, enemas or colema board sessions, especially at the very least just as you go into labour, to help side-step any unpleasant incidents during the birthing process… ;)

Transition

The phase of labour known as "Transition" is often experienced as the most intense part of the process, by many women. This stage involves the full dilation of the cervix to 10cm, just before the intense urge to push comes in. According to Ina May Gaskin, this is the critical point at which women often feel that they are not going to be able to go through with labour – they feel they are going to split apart and die. Ina recommends having someone around at this key juncture whom the birthing woman trusts, to assure the woman that the baby *is* going to ultimately come out, one way or another, that she is *not* going to split in half and that she *can* do this. Remember: this too shall pass ;)

Personally I don't recall the Transition stage of labour specifically – it didn't stand out to me… I was definitely very glad to have Ina May's wise words guiding me internally though… I also recalled a story she shared in one book of a woman she had encouraged by suggesting her body was going to be able to open up hugely to let the baby out. The woman really took on this idea and made it her birthing mantra: "I'm going to get huge". Sure enough, she easily opened out to release her big baby safely and swiftly – I appreciated recalling this story and mantra during birthing too, to help with my own opening process. Ina also thoroughly encourages women to keep their mouths and throats *open* as much as possible during labour, to keep the energy flowing and open, rather than tensed up and stuck.

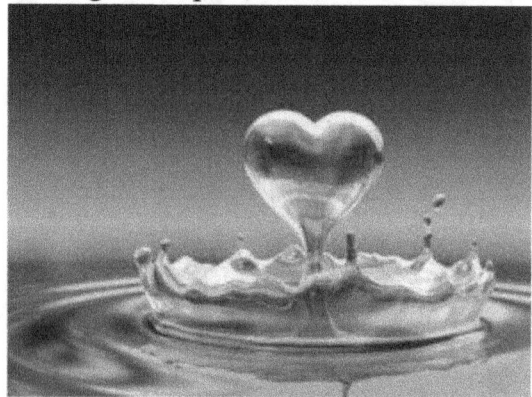

Why Water Birth?

Oria was birthed gently into our bath at home. There are many reasons people choose to give birth in water, including:

*natural pain relief

*warm water is soothing, comforting

*ease of movement

*gentle transition for baby from womb

*faster, less painful births on average

*natural buoyancy, woman feels lighter

*promotes deeper relaxation

*warm water softens body tissues, resulting in less tearing of perineum

*gentler, less stressful birth for the baby

For us it was an obvious choice to do a water birth and I would highly recommend it to any other woman, especially in terms of the natural pain relief. See waterbirth.org for lots of great information on birthing in water.

Lotus Birth

We did a lotus birth with Oria, meaning that we left the umbilical cord and placenta attached to her until they naturally dried up and detached by themselves, from the navel. There are many reported benefits of leaving a baby attached to their placenta, at least for a few hours after birth, if not a "full" lotus, where the cord and placenta are left to detach fully in their own time (usually 3-7 days after birth). People usually report that lotus babies are happier, seem more relaxed, more at ease in their bodies, cry less, don't get jaundiced as much, seem more connected to Spirit/Source, get all of the nutrition/nourishment possible from their placenta, tend not to lose weight in the first few days after birth like most babies and so on. To us it made sense to leave Oria with her placenta until they were both ready to let go.

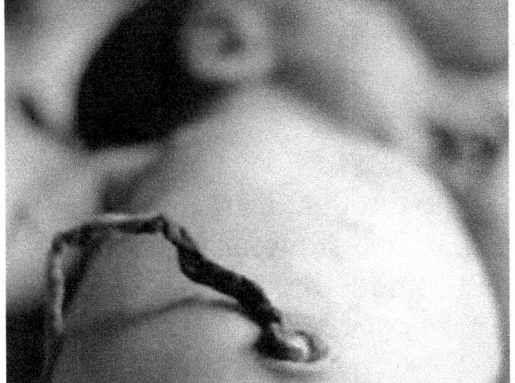

We kept the placenta in a little basket alongside Oria most of the time, bundled in a towel, though in the last day or so we started to keep it simply wrapped in a thick cloth, as this began to feel easier. At that point, we would bundle the placenta, wrapped in its cloth, against Oria's belly and wrap her up in a swaddling blanket. The placenta was kept salted and covered in herbs: lavender and rosemary oil, plus powdered nutmeg. Having the placenta still attached helped us to be extremely mindful and present when interacting with Oria and especially when moving her around.

It was amazing to watch the cord dry up from this thick blue-ish rope-like state to a thin, brittle sinew-like attachment that released almost precisely four days to the minute after Oria's birth. Our little girl was fully "Earthside". It was nice to not have the cumbersome cord/placenta/basket arrangement with her anymore.

At her navel she now had a perfectly-formed little belly button, which we treated with fresh aloe vera and breastmilk for the first few days, to help it fully heal. Apparently the falling off of umbilical stumps usually takes much longer than four days, for babies who are separated from their placenta at birth and left with a cord stump.

We took the released placenta, sliced it, dried it in the dehydrator, pulverised it, then encapsulated it as medicine for both Oria and I to potentially use for the rest of our lives. I put the capsules in the freezer to help preserve them for as long as possible and I take some whenever I feel drawn.

Oria Berry Monarch

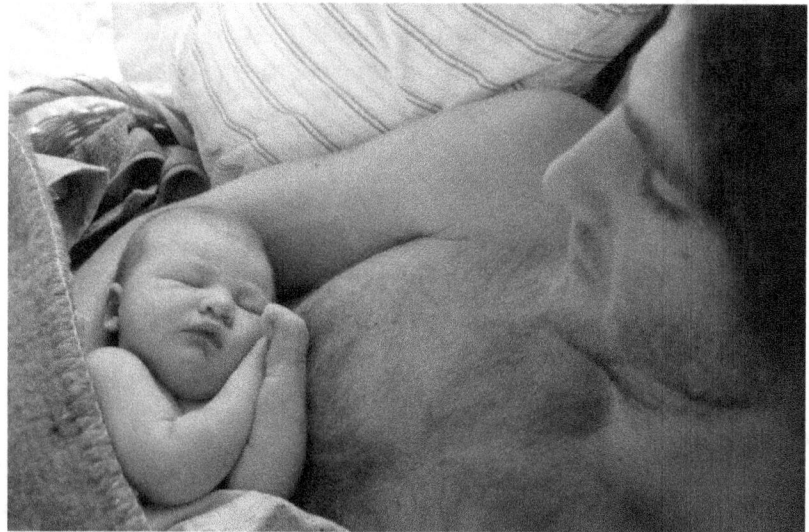

Oria chose her own first name and told Mr. M when she was a few days old… He was walking around with her and suddenly felt the name come through; he mentioned it to me, we both liked it and so it stuck. It was actually really interesting for us, as all through pregnancy I had been feeling the name "Soria" coming through for the baby, yet resisting it, as this happens to be the surname of a friend and we didn't want to be reminded constantly of someone else when saying our baby's name. Well, I guess I was just hearing an extra "S" at the start of the word, as Oria was the choice in the end ;) Another interesting aspect for us of this name game was that after we'd agreed on her name, a few days later I glanced over a list of possible baby names we'd been compiling throughout pregnancy and lo-and-behold, there it was: "Oria", in this very list. Somehow it just hadn't stood out to us until she was actually here, then it all fell into place – fascinating…

The name Oria seems to have two roots: Latin (Golden) and Hebrew (Light of God), so…putting it all together, she is seemingly the *Golden Light of God* :)

Berry has been a traditional middle name in my family since the 1700s… and then she is of course a Monarch, so… Oria Berry Monarch it is…

Doulas/Midwives

If we had not been able, for some reason, to have an unassisted birth as we intended, my next choice of "birthing style" would have been to have a female doula or midwife present with us, at home. I would prefer to have someone involved who is as "hands-off" as possible, with no internal examinations. Many women say that they find it extremely reassuring to have another woman there with them, especially one who has experience and insight to share in the area of childbirth.

If I were to search for a doula or midwife, I'd likely either ask for local recommendations in the area I was in, or otherwise consider bringing someone in from another area whose energy I feel I can connect well with. The energy, perspective and communication style of the people present at the birth can have *huge* effects in terms of how relaxed everyone is, how fast the labour goes, how much pain the woman experiences and so on – so choose your birthing companions *very* carefully indeed… ;)

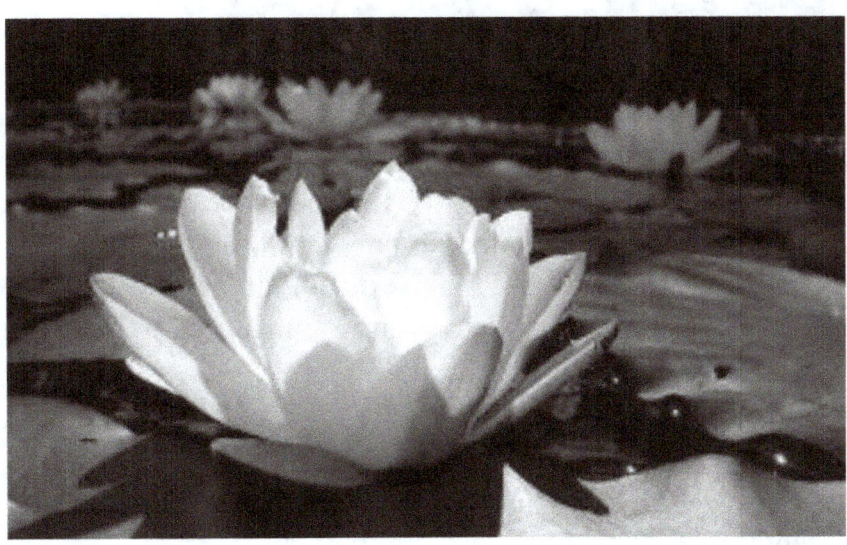

Post-Partum

Baby Moon

Immediately after Oria's birth, we began our "Baby Moon", wherein we posted notices on the outside of our house letting people know that we'd just welcomed a baby into the world and would appreciate time alone with her now for at least a week to allow for healthy bonding, rest and relaxation. This felt like such a kind gift to ourselves, as new parents often get overwhelmed in those opening days with all the integration that is unfolding in their family life, *plus* dealing with well-meaning, excited visitors day after day. We didn't want to add any extra pressures to our lives, so, up went the Baby Moon announcements and we settled into bed for peaceful bonding, rest and baby-gazing by the hour...

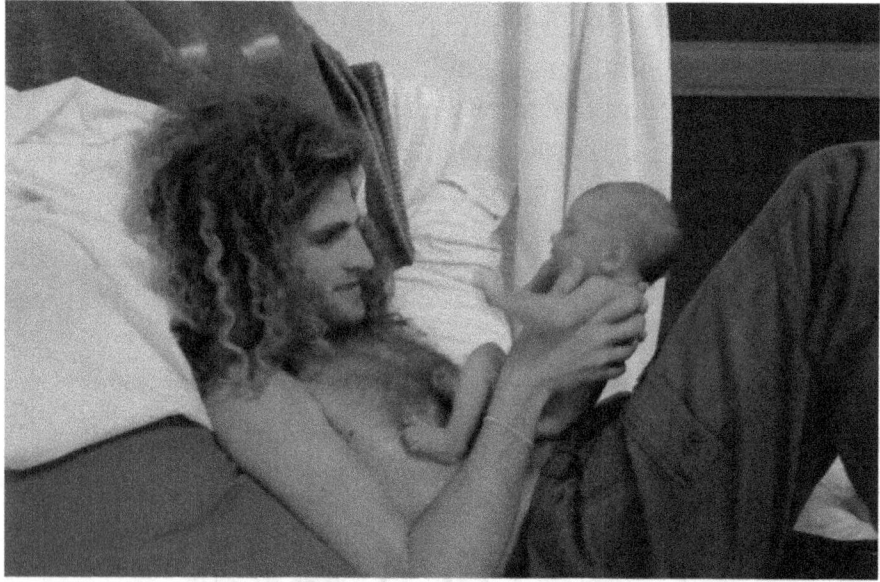

I would highly recommend "Baby Mooning" to other new parents. If people want to come by to *help* you with laundry or cleaning or food prep and so on, of course that's great, however, you might want to still make your boundaries very clear in terms of how long they stay, what they do and so on, until you're ready to be around more people again...

"Attachment" Parenting

Many of the practices we are enjoying with Oria come under the umbrella term of "Attachment Parenting", though not everyone likes that term... Some people prefer terms like "natural parenting", "conscious parenting" and so on... Whatever you choose to call it, here are some aspects of the life we choose to live with our baby:

Breastfeeding

Oria and I had some challenges getting our breastfeeding life together started. She was having a lot of issues trying to latch on and I was getting concerned that she was not feeding well. Fortunately we were very blessed to have wonderful friends right next door who came by to help us with getting things flowing. Katrina and Rineke came by, like our angel life-savers and sat with us for *hours* giving guidance, answering questions and helping us to get a good latch in place. As we got things going, my nipples became extremely painful in those first few days, cracked, bleeding, so sore…I would literally be crying putting Oria to the breast, as it was so painful, yet I knew that the only way onwards was to keep going through the pain. I had been forewarned by many women that the first couple of weeks of breastfeeding are typically very painful and to do my best to prepare the nipples in advance. Following this guidance, I had actually practiced nipple stimulation every single morning of pregnancy *(it's nice to get an oxytocin boost each morning as a side-effect too ;)*, however, I was still in agony post-partum. I used "Natural Nipple Butter" from Earth Mama Angel Baby almost constantly to help ease the pain.

A few weeks post-partum, someone asked me if I'd prepared my nipples during pregnancy using a *wire scrubber*…eeeeeeeek ;) I guess that's what some women do…and though I'm not sure I'd want to do that personally, I'd definitely encourage any pregnant woman to do as much as you can to toughen your nipples in advance, if you intend to breastfeed – you will SO appreciate it once the baby is here. *(Note: nipple stimulation in the very late stages of pregnancy might not be the best idea unless you're totally ready for the baby to arrive, as nipple stimulation is one of the things that helps to bring on labour…)*

Your nipples are also likely to change dramatically in appearance from breastfeeding. When I first saw breastfeeding friends' nipples, I was shocked – they were so *elongated* – about three times the length of a usual erect nipple, it seemed. I guess this comes from endless hours of being sucked on ;) I have since been told though that they usually return to pre-feeding size after weaning…

Once we got past those initial painful days and my nipples toughened up more, things started to feel easy with breastfeeding and it has remained that way since, I'm very happy to say. Oria *loves* to feed and would seriously feed 24/7 if she could, I think…she seems very orally fixated, with a strong sucking reflex and *loves* being latched on. I love seeing the crazy oxytocin-high "drunk" faces she produces when feeding: smiling, eyes rolling around, so content.

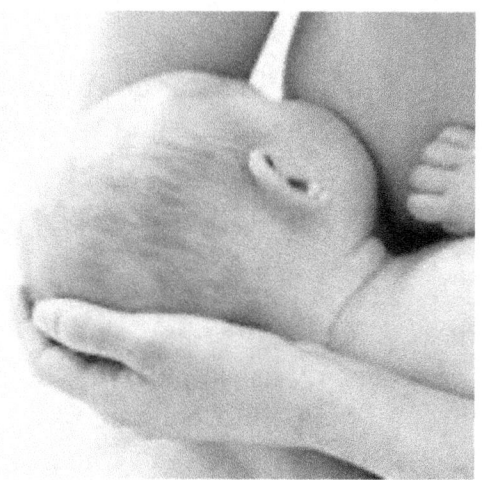

I would encourage any woman having issues with breastfeeding to connect with others for support, whether that's other breastfeeding mamas in your area, a La Leche League group or even just other people online. There are very useful breastfeeding videos, for example, on Dr. Jack Newman's site, http://www.breastfeedinginc.ca - you can watch video examples of good latches, poor latches, how to compress to get more milk flowing and so on.

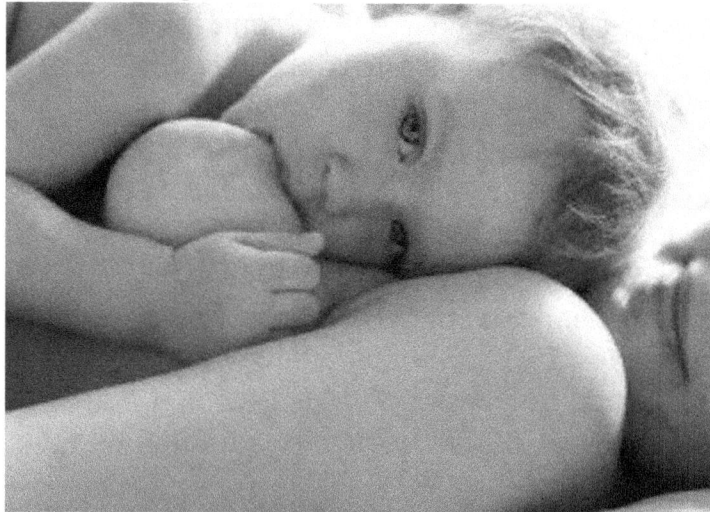

It is my intention to breastfeed Oria - and any subsequent siblings that may come along - for as long as they still want to feed. Some people call this "child-led weaning" or "full-term breastfeeding" and it's not uncommon for children fed this way to still be breastfeeding at least a couple of times daily at ages 4, 5, 6 or even 7 years, often in tandem with their younger siblings...left to their own flow and choices, children clearly seem to love and appreciate the nourishment and comfort of breastfeeding.

Oria is "exclusively" breastfed, on demand, at this point, meaning that she only consumes breast milk, nothing else, not even water and I feed her whenever she expresses hunger (See section on "Dunstan Baby Language, below). In terms of introducing solids, we also intend to follow Oria's lead, watching for when she starts to show interest in things other than breastmilk (tends to usually be somewhere around six months or so, from what I understand). At that point we will likely start her off with simple, soft raw foods such as avocado, papaya, mango and so on and take it from there…

You may find that you require a whole new set of clothes for breastfeeding, depending on your pre-pregnancy wardrobe…I personally found that I chose to only wear bamboo clothing in the first couple of months post-partum. Especially in the first weeks, my nipples were *so* incredibly sore that I couldn't bear for almost anything to touch them – bamboo felt like the softest, kindest choice in terms of clothing. I mostly have bamboo tops and dresses from the company Yala, in all kinds of styles appropriate for breastfeeding – i.e. easy breast access. You may also like to ensure you have *lots* of appropriate clothing available, especially if you intend to practice "Elimination Communication" (see below), as there are likely to be many "accidents" in the first months that end up on your clothing, plus of course spit-up, vomit and so on… ;)

Benefits of Breastfeeding

To me it's blatantly obvious that breastfeeding is the healthiest, clear choice for nourishing an infant, just like all mammals feed their young. However, let's go over some of the myriad benefits of breastfeeding here, just in case anyone is not quite on board yet:

*breastmilk is what baby humans are designed to consume – it is easy to digest and nutrient-packed.
*there's no financial cost.
*breastfeeding facilitates more physical contact and intimate bonding between mother and child.
*colostrum (first milk) contains nutrients and antibodies to build baby's immune system and protect them from illnesses.
*breastfed babies get ill less often on average.
*breast milk changes in response to the baby's requirements.
*breast milk is always ready, at the right temperature, with no equipment to prepare.

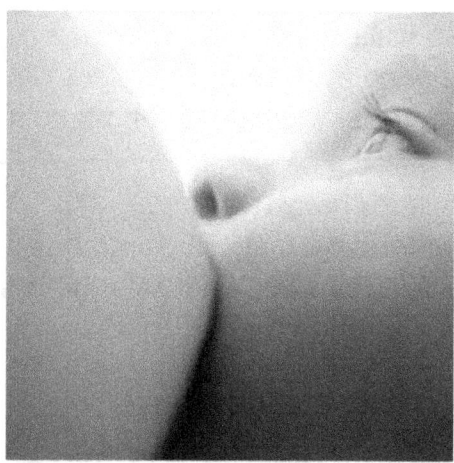

*breastfeeding involves significantly less environmental impact than bottle-feeding formula.

*breastfeeding can greatly reduce risk for baby of developing conditions such as asthma, diabetes, infections, allergies, obesity, SIDS and much more.

*breastfeeding also lowers the risk for the mother of developing many health conditions such as: diabetes, breast/ovarian cancer, postpartum depression, anemia, osteoporosis.

*promotes healthy facial structure/teeth development for baby, plus enhanced speech and visual development.

*on average, breastfed infants develop higher IQs, and have improved brain and nervous system development.

*breastfeeding helps the womb to contract back down after birth to control postpartum bleeding.

*breastfeeding acts like a natural contraceptive, delaying the return of the mother's menstrual cycle.

*the oxytocin released during breastfeeding helps both mother and baby feel calm, relaxed and connected.

*nursing mums usually get more sleep than formula-feeding mums.

…and this list could truly go on and on…as I said, for me, breastfeeding is the *obvious* choice for feeding an infant…I hope it is for you too.

Itchy Nose

One curious thing for me about breastfeeding, especially in the first weeks, was that I would suddenly get an *insanely* itchy nose, as soon as I started to feed Oria. So itchy that it would take *all* of my attention for a number of seconds… I tried researching the reason for this online and although I found many other women mentioning the same issue, I found no explanation for this strange phenomenon. As I write this, Oria is three months old and I still experience this itchy-nose phenomenon a little, however nowhere near as intensely as in those opening weeks…

Liquid Love

Drinking plenty of fluids seems to be key for both birthing women and breastfeeding mamas. I had plenty of fluids on hand during birthing, like coconut water and herbal tea (red raspberry with nettle). Then once Oria was Earthside, my desire for liquids was voracious, which is typical for breast-feeding mamas. Coconut water felt particularly nourishing for me in the first days after birth. In terms of post-partum herbal teas, a friend highly recommended drinking catnip tea to help side-step "colic"-y issues. I also love to make up my own herbal tea blends with different "carminative" (gas-reducing/expelling) herbs, such as: chamomile, fennel, lemon balm, red clover, peppermint, dill, anise, cumin, caraway. Great herbal teas for helping increase milk production include: raspberry leaves, nettles, alfalfa, red clover, borage leaves, fenugreek, plus blessed thistle tincture and fresh vegetable juices are extremely helpful too, especially carrot/green juice, apparently.

It's a very wise practice to try to always have plenty of liquid ready and available for you wherever you are breastfeeding. Also note that if your baby's soft spot/fontanel on their head is deeply depressed, they are very likely dehydrated, so pay attention to baby's fontanel and keep up that liquid love…

Co-sleeping

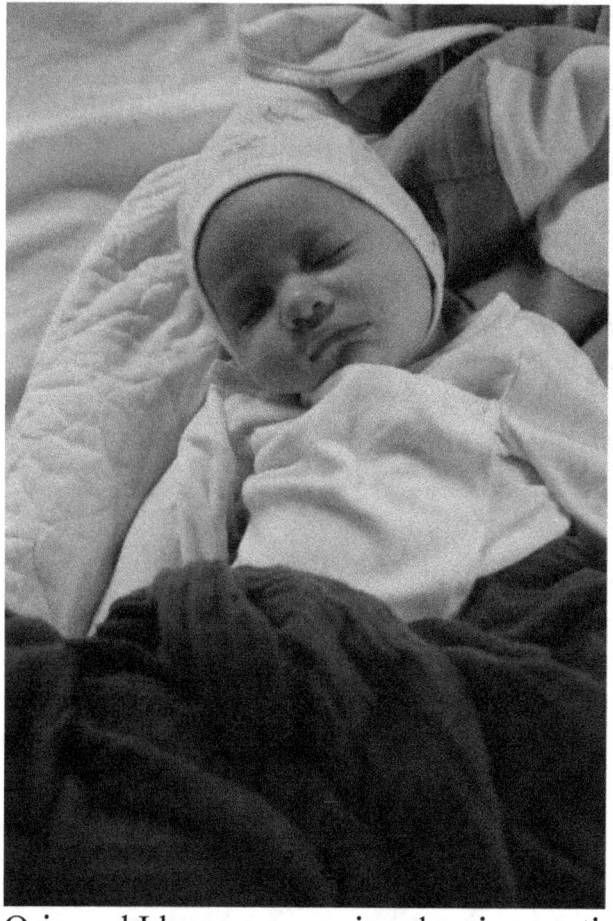

Oria and I have a very nice sleeping routine together, however, it didn't always feel that way…the first three weeks post-partum felt extremely challenging to me, with intense sleep deprivation. I have pretty much always slept on my front and now there was a co-sleeping baby here, who I wanted to be able to feed easily and keep in physical contact with me…and so I didn't know what to do anymore in terms of how to sleep. Laying on my back felt extremely unnatural and uncomfortable to me. Eventually we found a great solution. I piled a mass of pillows into the corner of the bed, against the wall and laid back into that, supported at an angle. Oria sleeps on her side, horizontally across my chest, supported by one of my arms wrapped along her back, plus our nursing pillow set behind her. Her face is aligned to either one of my nipples and she usually feeds as long as she wants, then pulls her head up and sets it back down again, using the breast as her pillow (so sweet ;) As I write this, Oria is a little over three months of age and we seem to now be slowly shifting into the next phase of this sleeping puzzle. Often now once she's asleep, I get to lay her down next to me and get some of that precious front-sleeping time for myself – bliss… Then when she wakes up to feed again (usually every three hours or so at this point), we shift back into the pillow pile and off we go again…

Personally I find it hard to believe that people who put their babies in another room to sleep are able to maintain sanity. It seems like disastrously more work to me, to get up, go into another room, change the baby, feed the baby, burp them, get them back to sleep, then go back to your own room to sleep…and to do this routine multiple times per night…this seems like a recipe for insanity to me; after all, sleep deprivation is a well-known form of torture… I feel extremely blessed that Oria and I have been able to settle into a pattern that keeps us close and seems to serve us both well in terms of getting good rest. It is actually amazing to me how she seems to just *know* that when we go to our outside bedroom at night, it's time for bed and we're into that three-hour feeding pattern with blessed sleep in-between… *(We sleep in a grounded, circular outside room made with just screen for walls and a glass roof, so that we have maximum airflow and can see the night sky, without being inundated with bugs…and horses ;)*

Mr. M has also been getting great sleep, in fact ever since Oria was born, his sleep has been disturbed very little. It seemed important to me for at least *one* of us to still be sane, so we left him to sleep as he always has and Oria and I had our own little night-time dance to unfold together. There's really nothing much he could even help with in the night, as the main thing she wants is to breastfeed, then go back to sleep, so there seems no point in disturbing his rest. This way he was also more able to hold space for us in those first few rollercoaster weeks when everything felt pretty intense for me in my hormonal-rollercoaster-sleep-deprived world…

We intend to co-sleep with Oria and any subsequent children who may come our way for as long as they want to sleep in the same bed as us, then we'll aim to help them set up whatever sleeping arrangement they would love…

Noisy Naps

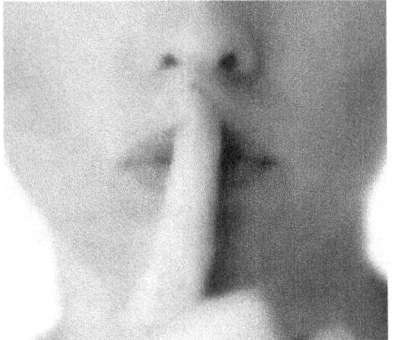

On the subject of sleeping, you might like to aim to establish from the very beginning what kind of noise levels you'd like your baby to be able to handle while sleeping. Babies tend to adapt to whatever we expose them to, so it could be in everyone's best interest if, rather than tip-toeing around your slumbering little one and trying to maintain silence, you just go about your life more-or-less as usual and help them to get used to sleeping in any context. I sense this is a much more valuable gift for a person in the long-run, to be adaptable with sleeping arrangements.

When Oria was first born, for some reason Mr. M and I both automatically started to speak the entire time in whispering voices...after a couple of days we suddenly realised what we were doing and that maybe this wasn't the best idea, as we surely didn't want to end up whispering for the rest of her infancy ;) So we started to talk at a standard volume and to go about life again more-or-less as usual, even when she's sleeping – this seems like a much wiser move overall, for us.

Bright Light, Bright Light

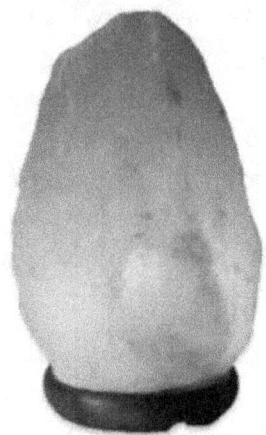

Babies are extremely sensitive to bright lights when they are first born, after just passing the last nine months or so in the cozy darkness of the womb. It's vital to protect their little eyes from bright lights in their opening days here. One suggestion we found especially useful in this regard was to use a beautiful salt lamp as the only lighting in the room we were in. The soft, warm amber glow of the salt lamp was gentle enough for Oria's little eyes to handle, while providing enough lighting for us at night to be able to take care of her safely. Plus of course the lamp also gives off wonderful, healthy negative ions constantly into our atmosphere – nice.

Baby-Wearing

Another "attachment parenting"-style practice we are engaged in is often called "baby wearing" or "continuum concept"-style parenting and basically involves having the baby in-arms/on your body as much as possible for the first months of life, usually up to at least a year or so in age. People often carry or "wear" their babies in slings, wraps or other baby carriers, to keep them close. The work of author Jean Liedloff is highly influential in this area, through her classic book "The Continuum Concept". Jean was extremely blessed to pass quite some time with a native tribe in South America, where she witnessed first hand how simple and yet remarkable the relationships there were between people, especially in terms of baby/child care. One of the main things she observed among these happy, healthy people was that they kept their babies in arms for the first year or so of life and hence she passed this on as a recommendation for helping babies in *our* societies feel more connected and at ease.

The first three months of a baby's life are often referred to as the "fourth trimester", as our infants, unlike so many other mammals, are *so* dependent when they're born – it's almost like caring for a fetus for the first few months. Unlike a baby giraffe, deer or horse, who can get running almost straight out of the womb if necessary, our babies are born "prematurely", in a sense, to be able to get our big heads and brains out of the birth canal. Keeping that dependent little one warm, close to you and feeling safe can really help in terms of bonding and development for your child. Remember, they were constantly enveloped by you 24/7 for nine months in utero, so even half an hour without touch can seem unbearable for a tiny new baby. Being left on their own in the wild could easily equal death for a tiny infant, so they definitely seem to prefer being held as much as possible in those opening months. It is also well known that babies in orphanages who do not receive plenty of human touch often die – loving touch is a *vital* part of the picture for our little ones.

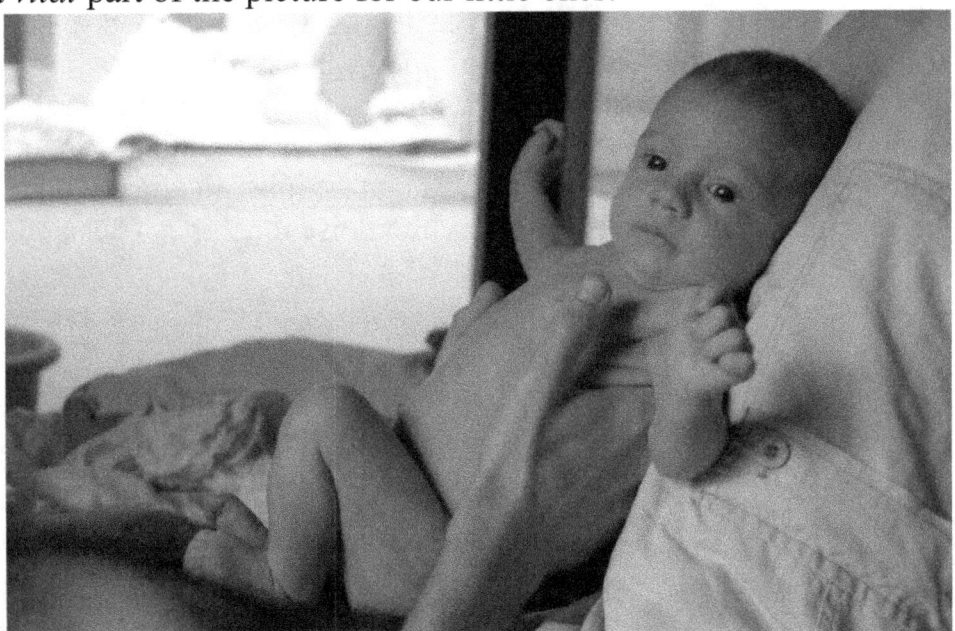

Skin-to-skin contact is especially nourishing for little ones and helps to regulate their body temperature too; babies can easily get cold in their first weeks of life, so it's great to have them with you skin-to-skin, or to make sure they're at least well dressed, especially wearing a little hat at night for example, as a great deal of body heat can be released via the head.

We almost always have Oria either in our arms or wrapped onto us with a Moby Wrap. We also have a sling, which we started to be able to use around two months of age, as she got head control then and it felt so much safer than when she was a floppy newborn. *(I was **so** happy when she got head control – it makes a **huge**difference in terms of moving her around… ;)*

I know many parents try out *multiple* wraps, slings and carriers over the months and years to see what feels best…both babies and caregivers can have different preferences and the best carrier for the job can change over time too. We have a "Boba" organic carrier ready for when Oria is older as well.

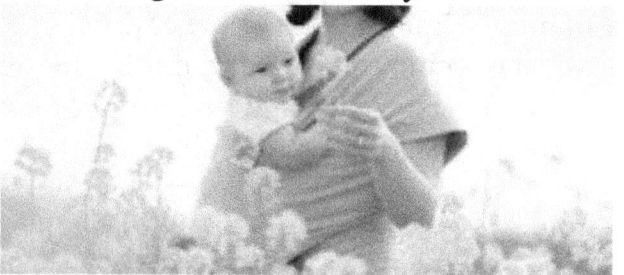

Oria is very happy being held/carried/in contact so much. When we wrap her up against us in the Moby Wrap she often fusses for a few minutes, then calms down totally and is usually asleep within another few minutes. She is very snugly held against us in the Moby, emulating the snug, warm confines of life in the womb, which makes it very comforting for such a young child. The easiest way I have found to help soothe her and get her to sleep is to have her Moby wrapped against me and to walk/jiggle around right next to our stone-grinder machines as they run, making raw nut/seed butters for us. Babies usually *love* white noise, as again, it emulates their experiences in the womb. Other "white noise" producers that people often use with babies include washing machines/dryers, hair dryers, white noise machines/CDs and so on…

Massage/Conscious Touch

Another key part of attachment parenting is to share loving, conscious touch with infants – one of the ways we do this daily with Oria is through gentle baby massage. Infant massage with healthy oils has a long history in Asian cultures and countless reported benefits, including:

*fostering bonding between caregiver and child
*calming
*neurological development
*colic relief
*sensory integration
*support for nervous system, digestion and musculo-skeletal system
*more rapid brain cell development, as oils applied directly to scalp penetrate through and feed the brain.

It's remarkable to me that a simple, enjoyable little ten-minute massage with Oria each day can bring so many benefits for her. We personally use the outrageously fabulous Andreas' Oils on Oria's skin – the White Sesame is my favourite so far for working with her. I especially concentrate on getting plenty of oil onto her head and back daily, to help assist her brain and spinal development. I just smooth the oil gently all over her, being careful not to apply much pressure, especially not on the soft spots on her head of course. She seems to *love* massage and I am very happy to be able to share this with her daily.

Elimination Communication

Oria is a "nappy/diaper-free" baby. We are following the practice of "Elimination Communication" (EC) wherein we are learning to communicate together about when she wants to go to the toilet and helping her to release over a bowl, potty, toilet or other receptacle, rather than into her clothing, which would otherwise then be held against her body. She wears no nappies/diapers, just standard clothing. This is a traditional practice for people all around the world and the benefits are myriad: we can work with the child from birth to help them keep themselves clean, rather than leaving them to soil themselves daily for a couple of years before "toilet training"; we can develop strong bonding and communication together from tuning in to each others' messages, we can help the child have more trust in us to help them and more confidence in their own bodies, we can drastically decrease the environmental impact of using nappies/diapers, whether disposable or cloth, we can dramatically reduce the financial cost of child-raising and so on.

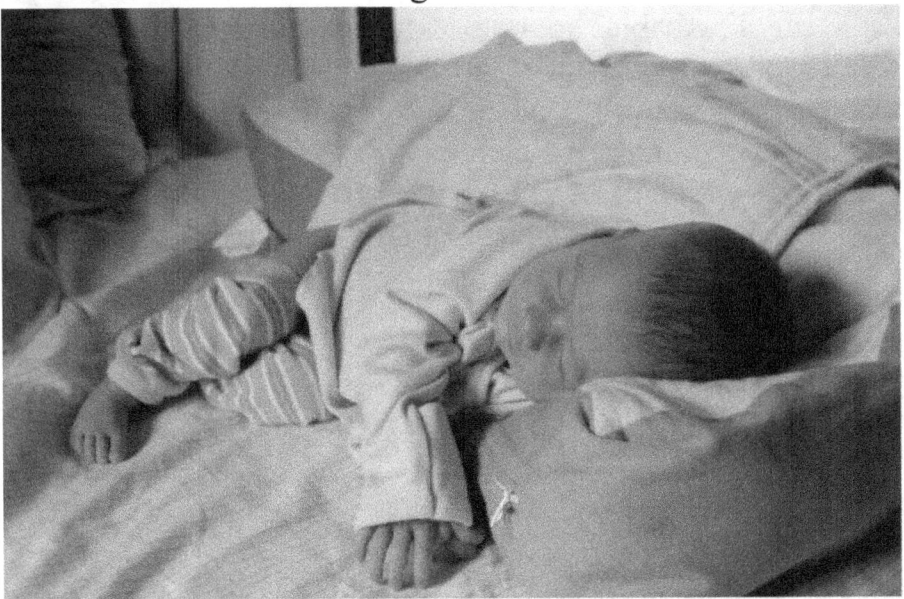

There are various ways that people communicate with their babies about toilet requirements: some people go by the facial expressions or gestures of the baby, some go by timing, some "cue" the baby with sounds when they feel it's time, some go by intuition and so on. Many people use a combination of these techniques, us included. Personally at this point I tend to go mostly by timing: I simply think to myself "it's been a while since she last went" and I hold her over the plastic box we usually use to catch her deposits and see if she wants to go or not. I use a "pssssssssss" sound to cue her to urinate and a deep grunting noise to cue a bowel movement. I hold her with her back resting against my torso, with one of my hands supporting her under each of her legs, in a kind of seated position over the box. We use a fairly large plastic box with a lid, so that we can contain the smell and avoid unwanted spills. I notice that she urinates a lot usually in the mornings, perhaps every thirty minutes or so, then the pace tails off over the day.

Oria almost always wants to urinate immediately after waking up, so that's always an easy one to catch. She also at this point tends to want to do a bowel movement after waking up from a long sleep; so first thing in the morning and after sleeping in the middle of the day I check to see if she also wants to release a bowel movement after waking. She tends to get a very interesting look of concentration on her face when she wants to do a bowel movement and makes some low grumbling noises, so it is often quite easy to tell when she wants to go.

We started EC when Oria was around three weeks of age, as prior to that I simply felt too overwhelmed with everything else we were learning to start practicing it. We were very blessed to have good friends living nearby who had practiced EC with their four-year-old daughter. One day in Oria's third week, they were visiting and helped us to get going with EC by simply holding Oria over a little bowl, cueing her with the psssssssss sound and…voila…from the very first attempt, she responded immediately :) It was amazing to me – it's truly like babies are born with the "programme" to respond in this way. Most EC babies are fully toilet independent by 18 months or so of age, whereas most babies in general have not even *started* "toilet training" by that age. Many EC babies communicate extremely efficiently with their caregivers about their toilet requirements at just a few months of age – babies do not *want* to soil themselves and sit in their own waste any more than we adults do…

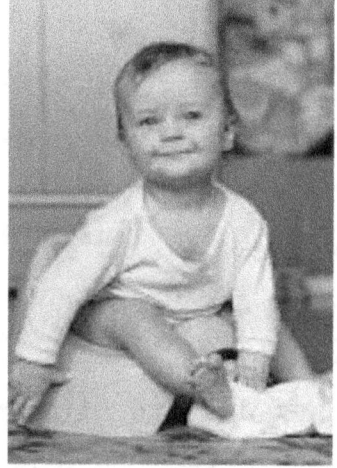

The biggest concern that people usually have about EC is: what happens if you "miss" a deposit…? For us this has never been a concern…we live in a house with tile floors, we have plastic mattress covers on the beds and plenty of clothes to change both Oria and ourselves into if we get wet or stained. We choose not to create "drama" if we miss one of Oria's eliminations – we do not choose to perceive it as an issue - yet I can understand though that not everyone may feel relaxed with such "accidents". Whatever you choose to do, I would strongly suggest treating your child always with love, affection and compassion as you clean them up and change their clothes, to help them feel good about their bodily functions, rather than potentially going into feelings of shame or discomfort. They are learning how to be in this new body and in time they will surely be very efficient at keeping themselves clean and dry.

As I write this, we've been practicing EC with Oria for about two and a half months and we easily catch the vast majority of her deposits now and have done so for weeks. She actually holds urine in already and waits until we have her in position to release. It's quite remarkable and yet of course at the same time, totally natural and common worldwide – it's just *us* in our so-called "civilised" societies who usually work with such a strange alternative system of nappies/diapers. I'm personally extremely happy to not be part of that system and I'm sure Oria is too…

The main resource we used to learn about EC was Ingrid Bauer's book "Diaper Free", which I'd highly recommend. There are other books, websites, online videos and DVDs out there you can explore too…

Things You Might Not Know About Life Post-Partum…

There are many things that happen after the baby is born that might be a bit of a surprise if you're not forewarned. Apparently it's extremely common that parents-to-be focus a great deal on *pregnancy and birthing* and very little on how life will be *post-partum*, once the baby is actually here… Yet as author Robin Lim reminds us, you're pregnant for only nine months and post-partum for the rest of your life. Here are some of the perhaps lesser-mentioned aspects of life immediately post-partum that come to my mind, which you might appreciate knowing about in advance…:

* **After-Birth Contractions** – nope, you're not done with contractions even after the placenta arrives… ;) The womb has a lot of work to now do to get back down to its pre-pregnancy size, so, following delivery of the placenta and in the days/weeks to come, you'll likely experience abdominal cramping, similar to menstrual cramps, especially whenever you nurse, if you're breastfeeding, as the uterus shrinks back down. For me these cramps and twinges did not feel very severe and tailed off completely somewhere around four weeks post-partum. You can assist this shrinking back down of the womb by regularly massaging your lower abdomen in the first days and weeks post-partum.

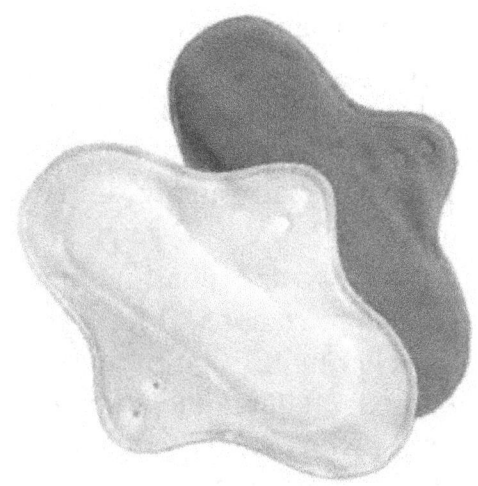

*Lochia – along with those after-birth contractions, you'll almost definitely have a pretty heavy amount of bloody discharge too, for the first few weeks postpartum; this is known as "lochia". This is another aspect of the womb clamping back down and clearing out any remaining debris. Expect something like a heavy, red menstrual flow in the first days, which usually then turns more brownish in colour after a while, then tails off. It's wise to have thick, absorbent menstrual pads on hand to deal with this outpouring.

*Hair Loss – this was a sad part of the picture for me… It is very common for women to lose a lot of hair post-partum. The reason for this is apparently because *usually* a small percentage of a non-pregnant woman's hair is "resting" (not growing), after which it falls out. During*pregnancy* however, one of the results of the changes in hormones is that this "resting then falling out" pattern goes on hold. People often comment on how lush, thick and healthy pregnant women's hair looks…*then*, post-partum, the hormones switch again and now there is a massive shedding, leaving your shower drains clogged, your hairbrush matted up like crazy and stray hairs wrapped all around your baby's fingers, if your house is anything like ours… There's nothing really to be done about this situation, other than just deal with all the extra hair all over the place…apparently within a year or so, most women's hair is back to how it looked pre-pregnancy.

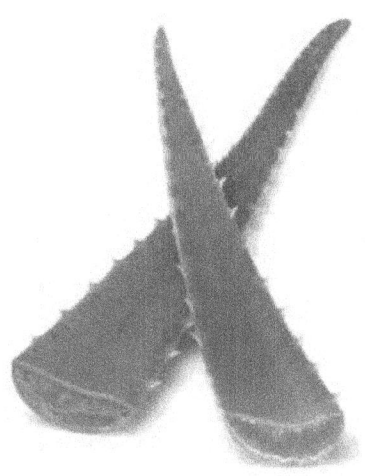

*Healing Tearing/Stitches – most women who birth vaginally find that their perineum either tears a little during childbirth, or, in a "medicalised" birth context, women often receive an episiotomy (wherein the perineum is *intentionally* cut open, to allow more room for the baby to emerge, then re-stitched afterwards – OUCH :O …) Either way, you're likely to have an extremely sensitive and delicate under-carriage for the first few weeks at least. At first I thought I hadn't torn, then after a few days I realised I actually had…fortunately, I'd been using aloe vera compresses from immediately after birth, so I had been assisting the healing process from the very beginning. I would highly *highly* recommend aloe compresses to any woman after birthing – I felt like the aloe was my saviour. We would take a big, thick leaf of fresh aloe, cut away the green outer skin, to reveal the thick juicy filet inside, then I would lay that filet on top of a cloth menstrual pad and press it all up to my skin. It felt so cooling and relieving and the most amazing part to me was that after a few hours, this thick juicy aloe filet would be shrunk down to a paper-thin state – my body was just *sucking* up all of the healing goodness from the plant and mending my tissues. I felt so immensely grateful. A friend later told me she did the same thing with the added step of *freezing* the aloe filets, so that they were extremely cooling and relieving next to her damaged tissues – "cool" idea ;)

It took me about four weeks post-partum to get to the point where it didn't hurt anymore to urinate and it seemed like things were more or less healed up. Many women do things like sitz baths, compresses and squirting warm water into their vaginal area with a squeezy bottle while urinating, to help ease the pain… I experimented with some of these other things, yet found the aloe filets to be my greatest ally.

It is also not recommended for women to take baths or open their legs much in those first few weeks of healing – there is so much adjusting for the body to do after opening SO wide to get that baby out. The opening through to the womb can still be somewhat open and there is a greater risk of infection in that area, so do your best to take things very easy in those opening days, to maximise your healing potential.

If you're keen to *avoid* perineal tearing, you might love to do your best to prepare your perineum in advance during pregnancy, by doing daily massage of the tissue there for example and doing kegel exercises (squeezing up the muscles of the undercarriage area). During birth you can also hold warm oil compresses against the area, have someone massage/support the area and aim to deliver the head sloooowly to help reduce sudden tearing – all of these can help preserve the integrity of the tissues.

*Baby Blues – almost all women (up to 80%, apparently) experience some "baby blues" as part of the hormonal, sleep-deprived rollercoaster of life post-partum. There can be intense, oxytocin-fuelled, blissed out highs and then crashing, deep, hysterical lows. Women are typically very weepy, emotional, anxious and sensitive at this time, often accompanied by self-doubt, insecurity and exhaustion. It can be quite a humbling experience – be sure to ask for and accept help and support wherever you can and to talk honestly with others about what you're experiencing, so that you keep your emotions flowing and don't feel stuck in your head.

Personally I was feeling so emotional in those first weeks that I couldn't even get through singing a single song to Oria – I'd start and within two lines I'd just dissolve into tears…everything seemed so poignant…

I think it's very wise to make sure that anyone around a newly post-partum mother *realises* about this pattern of extreme sensitivity, to try to make the situation as gentle and easy as possible for all involved. Any supportive, encouraging, affirming words shared with the new mama at this time are likely to be highly appreciated by her and can help her to feel more secure that she's doing a good job.

*Leaking Breasts – if you are breastfeeding, in the beginning you will almost certainly find that as you feed the baby on one side, the other breast leaks all over you. I used to position a little bowl underneath the leaking breast to catch the excess in the first few weeks. Breast milk is great for treating any skin issues, belly button healing, eye concerns and so on. After maybe the first four weeks or so, the leaking stopped for me and I was glad. I didn't do anything special to get the leaking to stop, it just happened by itself, though some women do use tricks like pushing up against the leaking breast with a fist to stem the flow.

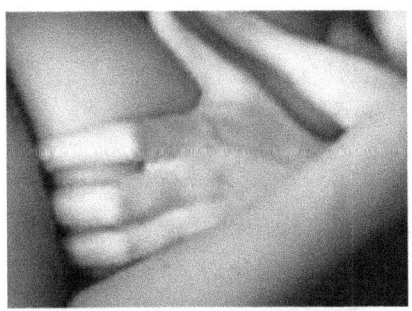

Incidentally, you might also find it useful to know in advance that babies' tiny little nipples also sometimes leak milk in the first days/weeks post-partum. Due to the influence of the mother's hormones, you might notice a tiny drop or two of milk leaking from your little one's nipples – this is nothing at all to be concerned about and is very common. We experienced this for a couple of days with Oria.

*The One-Handed Genie – if you intend to practice an "attachment" style of parenting, get used to doing a lot of things one-handed, or even no-handed at times (e.g. using your feet, elbows, teeth and so on to get things done…). Even when using slings or wraps to hold your baby, you often have only one hand free, while supporting the child with the other hand. You may discover a whole new depth of meaning to the expression "left holding the baby", once a little one is actually here in your hands… I often think it would have been a very useful evolutionary feat if these wild pregnancy-related hormones also led a woman to sprout an extra arm or two post-partum… ;)

Be prepared to *slooooooooooow dooooooown* – you cannot easily do things at a fast pace anymore, especially one-handed. This book is actually a prime example – it was typed out almost entirely one-handed, while supporting Oria with the other hand…

*Jaundice – the majority of babies become jaundiced after birth. This is due to an excess of bilirubin in their systems. Making sure you give the baby daily exposure to sunlight can help tremendously to clear this condition. Just 3-4 minutes of direct sunlight, or around 20 minutes of indirect sunlight per day can help clear things up in a week or so. Fortunately for us, Oria didn't deal with this condition. According to master herbalist Susun Weed, if the mother drinks dandelion root tea, this can also help the baby's liver develop and clear the jaundice faster.

*Meconium – your baby's first bowel movements, for the first few days, consist of a sticky blackish-greenish tar-like substance called "meconium". This stuff is often very sticky and messy, so you might like to make sure that in the beginning your baby has some piece of old clean cloth next to their bottom, or something you don't mind getting very dirty/stained, or even throwing away.

Interestingly, it seemed that Oria's meconium wasn't as "sticky" as many babies' and was easy to clean off her – perhaps this was in some way related to the fact that I eat raw bee-gan…?

*Weight Loss – most babies lose weight in their first few days Earthside – usually a few ounces and according to Ina May Gaskin, preferably no more than 10% of their original birth weight. This lost weight is usually regained within a couple of weeks and the child typically goes on gaining from there at a rate of around 6oz a week. This is very common, yet could be very concerning to a new parent if you didn't know. This was indeed the pattern that Oria followed, though we hear that many Lotus Birthed babies do *not* follow this weight loss pattern.

*Eye Issues – newborns often have gunky, crustie mucus deposits at the sides of their eyes. Most of these issues can be dealt with using simple, natural remedies, for example, a couple of drops of breastmilk in each eye, or a drop of colloidal silver, or a swab of chamomile tea.

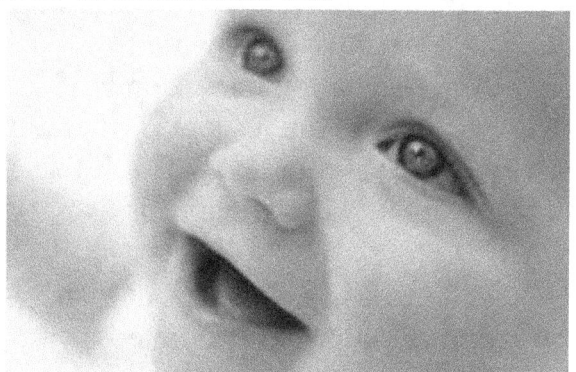

With Oria we had the added complication that the tear duct of her left eye was not open, another common issue with newborns. Usually tears move across the eyes to keep them lubricated and drain down the tear duct into the nose/throat area. When the tear duct is not yet open, the tears overflow out of the eye instead, leaving the baby with a constant accumulation of liquid at the inner side of the eye. Fortunately it's easy to help the tear duct to open with some simple, gentle massage at the inner corner of the eye – just a few days of massage was enough to help Oria's tear duct open. Babies often *appear* to be cross-eyed too from time to time when they are very young – don't panic. This is very common and nothing to be concerned about – the eyes just aren't fully coordinated yet; they are unlikely to stay that way… Many babies also apparently have small haemorrhages in their eyes after birth, due to the pressure of the birth canal – again, this is nothing to be concerned about and it will usually clear up in the first few days.

*Squishes – many babies are born with parts of their bodies "squished" up in some way or another…maybe one of their ears is folded over from the way they were wedged inside the womb, maybe their head bones got squished a little into an unusual temporary shape while they were coming through the birth canal, maybe their feet are squished in at a funny angle and so on. All of these kinds of things will straighten themselves out soon; there is no need to panic. The womb and birth canal are simply snug places to fit into for a full term baby, so these kinds of "squishes" are to be expected. When Oria arrived, I was very concerned that she had a "club" foot, as her right foot was held at such a curious, squished up angle, however she's totally fine now and it's straightened out…and I was also so concerned that she had a "lazy" right eye, until I realised it was just that she mostly laid on me on her right side, so that eye wasn't so easy to open ;) It can be very easy to have countless concerns about your little one once they're here, however, rest assured that most "squishes" tend to work themselves out – just give them time…

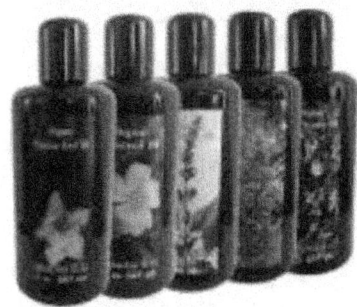

*Cradle Cap – it seems that most babies also get "cradle cap", a scaly, harmless build-up on their scalps that can be very challenging to remove. We felt very blessed to be able to pretty easily remove Oria's cradle cap at around two months of age. I do massage with her daily with Andreas' White Sesame Oil, especially focusing on her scalp. These daily massages seemed to help a great deal to soften up the cradle cap and then on a couple of occasions when she was particularly warm, it became very easy to just smear the cradle cap off her head – hurray :) I avoided removing the cradle cap from her soft spot/fontanel so far though, as I don't want to apply any pressure there.

*New Limits - once the baby is here with you Earthside, for at least the first few months, it is likely to feel very challenging to do many things for yourself that would have felt totally easy to engage in before. For example, cutting your toenails, getting your hair cut, watching a film without interruption, making a special meal, going on a leisurely trip to somewhere you want to go…all of these kinds of things and many many more can take on a whole new level of challenge with a newborn in your arms…

It's tough to imagine before your little one is actually here just *how* different your life is likely to feel…as one friend said to me "it's like there's nowhere *in* a person for this information to land until they actually become a parent – it goes in one ear and out the other, people just can't relate until their baby is actually here – and then it's too late!"

So, I believe it would be a very wise idea to do as many of the things for yourself that you'd love to do PRIOR to your baby's arrival, to avoid feelings of frustration…if there's some film you'd love to see, some restaurant you'd love to go to, some trip you've been longing to go on, consider doing these things BEFORE the baby is here, to avoid having built-up, unfulfilled desires rustling around in the back of your head for the first months of your baby's life.

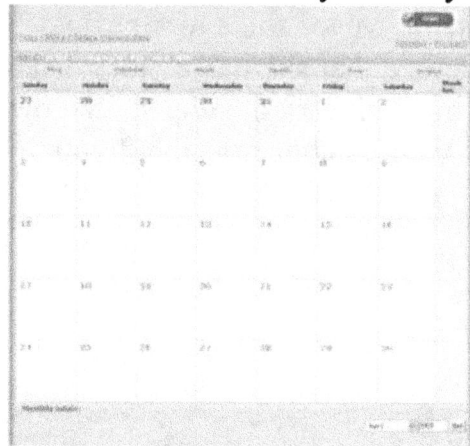

Now, this is of course not to suggest that once a baby is in your life, you become unable to do anything *you* want – that is not necessarily the case at all, I just want to share something of this pattern here to help people be at least a little more prepared for the reality of life with a newborn…

I would furthermore strongly recommend aiming to clear your schedule as *much* as possible from around your "due date" and onwards. I thought our baby was going to join us in December, so my calendar was basically blank from December onwards…I had no *real* idea what life was going to look like once the baby was here, yet I felt very strongly that I did not want to add even a *moment* of extra stress into my life through planned events on my schedule – maybe this resonates for you too…

Also, be aware that it's likely going to take a while to work out how to do things now with a baby at your side, e.g. going to the toilet, going shopping, preparing food, eating and so on. It might take a few weeks to adjust and find your new rhythms together, so, do your best during this period of adjustment to be *kind* to yourself, your baby and anyone else helping you, like your partner. This is new for all of you and doing your best to be supportive, gentle, patient, honest and compassionate at this time is likely to help make it easier for everyone. You'll work it all out soon enough, especially with careful observation of the baby to help determine faster your new rhythms together. This too shall pass…

*New Skills

It can feel like there's so much to *learn* with a newborn suddenly under your care. Suddenly trying to learn a whole new skill set *post-partum,* when you're quite likely already feeling exhausted, sleep deprived, anxious and insecure might not be the wisest way to go about things…

I would highly recommend trying to get some practice *before-hand* with skills you think will be useful, such as bathing a baby, swaddling, carrying a baby in a sling or wrap and so on. You might practice these things with a doll, ask to watch/participate with a friend who has a baby, or even just watch some videos online…the more insight and practice you can get before-hand, the easier it will hopefully be when you suddenly have a real life, floppy, screaming newborn in your hands ;)

A word of warning though: I'm not sure anything can *fully* prepare you for the reality of life with a newborn… I thought that Mr. M and I were particularly at a disadvantage in terms of our learning curve post-partum, as both of us had very little experience with babies prior to Oria arriving, however, I later spoke to a friend who was the eldest of eight children and had masses of baby-care experience in her life and she told me that she doesn't feel it really makes much difference – nothing could have prepared her for the reality of suddenly having her own tiny, writhing newborn in her hands to take care of, 24/7…

In terms of scaling the immense learning curve of parenthood, one of the kindest pieces of guidance that was shared with me at the very beginning was from an older friend who assured me that "we all make "mistakes"; it's part of the process, just keep doing your best." She shared an example with me of how she felt that she had almost accidentally drowned her oldest daughter as a baby when she was paying so much attention to washing her *feet* in the bath that she forgot to support her head from slipping underwater…the baby was fine of course and for me it was reassuring to hear this message that "mistakes" are to be expected along the way of this huge learning curve and to just keep on doing my best…

Prioritisation

One thing motherhood has definitely encouraged me further into is prioritisation. Motherhood is no place for procrastinators… Whenever I get a few precious minutes of time where I have both hands to myself and Oria is with someone else, I find myself rushing around, aiming to get as much done as I can while my hands are free…and the key for me is to *prioritise*– if there's something I really want done, then that's what I go to first, as I never know how long I'm going to have hands-free. This helps to keep me from procrastination and on a more efficient track, so I can really see it as a blessing in this way…

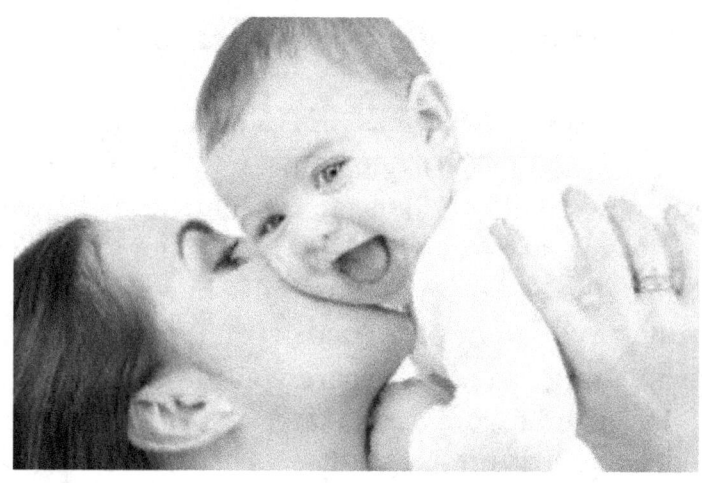

Surrendering the Self

As the saying goes, "there's no "I" in "we"" and when your little one comes along, you may feel this more keenly than ever. Human babies are extremely dependent when they're born – they would soon die without our help and it can feel, in the opening weeks especially, that your *own* self, as you have known it, is in fact "dying". You are no longer a singular unit – you have an offspring and that little being is looking to you in every moment of every day for love, support and compassion. A certain degree of surrendering your own "self" tends to unfold in the wake of the arrival of such little beings… Now, while *overstretching* yourself into an unhealthy, constantly child-centred reality is not likely the best idea, you *will* almost certainly find that things you want to do often end up going on hold, or not getting done at all, or maybe get done by someone else…living life focused almost exclusively focused on your *own* agenda isn't really gonna fly anymore…

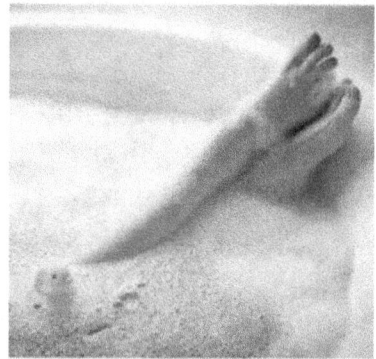

This all being said, I do feel that it is absolutely *key* for parents to take time, space and energy where we can to re-fill our own inner wells too: we can only give what we have. Do things that help you to feel open, loving, connected, happy…take that bath, call that friend, go for that walk…it is essential for *you* to be happy in order to show up as the best parent you can be for that tiny little button at your side…

Mama?

I have found it quite odd to start identifying *myself* with the term "mum" and the concept that *I'm* someone's parent (i.e. *"Me? A parent? How did that happen? That's a word that applies to other people, not me…" ;)*.

I experienced something similar after marrying – it felt very odd at first to adapt to a sudden reality shift that I was someone's "wife", I had a "husband" and I had even changed my name somewhat, adding on a "Monarch" to the end… Now I'm feeling the same way about being someone's "mum", though I'm *starting* to get used to it and maybe by the time Oria actually starts to call me "mama" I'll be used to the new label. ;)

Resting

It is absolutely vital for a new mama to get as much rest as she can in the first weeks after birth. The body is going through so many shifts and there is so much to learn… Accept all and any help you can get for those opening days and weeks, so that you can concentrate on bonding with your newborn – your most important task now. The laundry can be done by someone else, or it can wait – you will never again have these precious moments to bond with your little one and recuperate from the transition of birthing. Rest, rest, rest as MUCH as you can. It can be so tempting to run around constantly "getting things done", perhaps fuelled by post-birth euphoria, however, the more you can take things easy and rest at this point, the faster your overall healing can unfold. Be gentle with yourself, try to sleep when the baby sleeps and do *nothing* "extra", only the bare minimum of priorities to keep things flowing. One thing I found that I kept saying in the first few weeks of Oria's life was "I have no idea how single parents cope – or parents with multiple babies"… Kudos and highest blessings to all of you out there in those situations – it seems challenging enough just having *one* baby and a supportive partner…may you be surrounded with support and blessed with adequate rest…

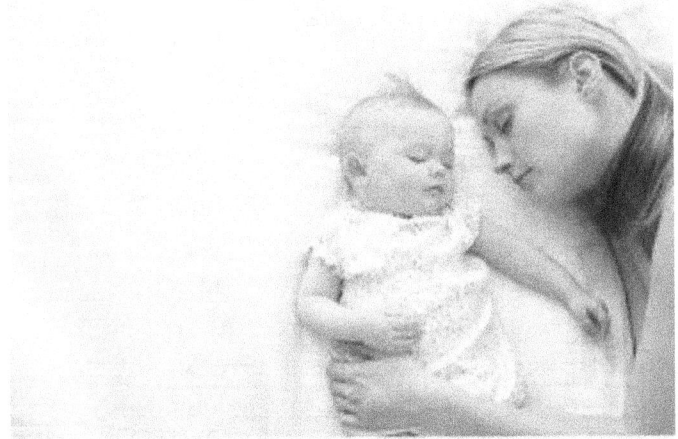

Many cultures around the world have traditions of new mamas resting for at least a certain number of weeks post-partum – it might be 40 days, 62 days, three months or six weeks; the number of days may differ, yet clearly it's a common pattern. Usually the new mama is supported to rest and heal as *much* as possible in this period, with lots of help for food preparation, cleaning, child care and so on. Personally I didn't go *anywhere* with Oria until she was five weeks old, which happened to be Christmas Day and we went to a friend's house for a little potluck party. Prior to that day I could not at *all* get my head around the idea of going anywhere with her and even on that day, taking her out in a car, being with her at a party, changing her clothing and feeding her in a different place all felt really bizarre. It was a very mellow party though, with sweet people and turned out to be a good first outing experience for us – it went really well and helped me feel confident to be able to go out to more places with her, though I was definitely grateful and glad for those first five quiet weeks at home we had enjoyed immediately post-partum and we certainly didn't rush into any hectic social schedule after five weeks either – a slow and simple lifestyle works best for us…

Chiropracty/Cranio-Sacral

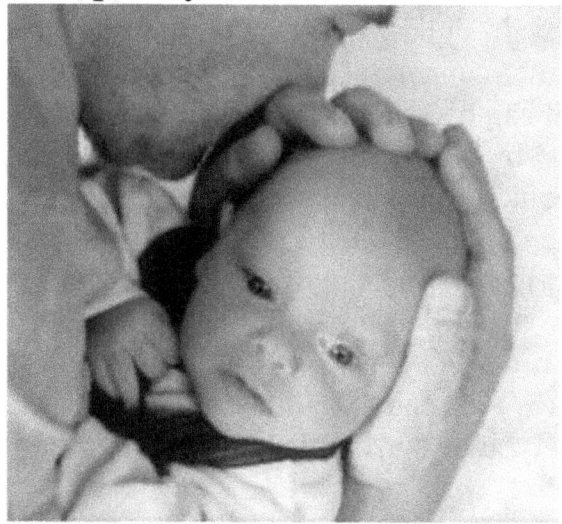

I would highly recommend having your baby checked out by a chiropractor, a cranio-sacral therapist, or anyone else who is familiar with the workings of the spine/head/spinal fluid. A simple adjustment for a baby who is holding themselves in even a slightly strange position can make a huge difference. I strongly remember a friend years ago with a baby girl who was crying a great deal. The mother intuitively sensed it had something to do with the way the baby was holding her back, after birth. She took the baby for a chiropractic session and *immediately* after the chiropractor worked on the baby's spine, she relaxed all over, gave a huge smile and ceased her painful screaming. For Oria, we had a fabulous body-worker friend check her out – he helped to release a little stiffness in her sacrum and other than that she was in great alignment, I am happy to say. A session of this kind is definitely something you might want to consider to help your little one get the best start in terms of their spinal alignment.

Soothing Baby

Oria doesn't cry much – mainly just in the early evenings so far (I suspect as a result of gas build-up in her body during the day), however, listening to that heart-wrenching sound moment-to-moment as it unfolds can feel very challenging. Like all babies, she always has a *reason* for crying of course, e.g. hungry, tired, over-stimulated, gas, too cold and so on – she wouldn't use her energy up on crying for "no reason", so it's a question of working out what she wants right then and helping her feel better. It's important to remember that as babies cannot yet speak, crying is one of their primary ways to let us know what is happening for them – it can sound *so* desperate and extreme and yet the situation is almost always quite easily resolvable if we can just determine what it is the baby is disturbed about and help soothe them.

The Dunstan Baby Language system has been indispensable for us in regards to working out what is happening for Oria. Developed by Priscilla Dunstan in Australia, the Dunstan system reveals that there are five distinct sounds that *all* newborn babies in the world make, regardless of their race, location, parents' language or any other factors. Each sound is connected to a natural reflex in the baby's body and each has its own meaning, related to what the baby wants to communicate. These five sounds are: "neh" for "hungry", "eh" for upper wind, "eairh" for lower gas, "owh" for tired and "heh" for uncomfortable. With Oria's voracious appetite, the sound we hear most often from her is "neh" – it is very distinct and this system has been incredibly useful for us in terms of helping to settle and soothe Oria, as we can quickly determine what it is that she wants.

Note though that your baby uses a lot of the same muscles to breastfeed and to cry…so if baby is at the point of *screaming* to be fed, even once you get them near the breast, it may take some time for them to actually get calm enough to take the nipple and start feeding; give them time and help to soothe them as best you can until they have calmed enough to feed. If after a few minutes they still haven't calmed enough to latch on, it's possible that they don't actually want to feed right then and there's something else to attend to for them – perhaps burping, peeing or changing their clothes, for example.

Another resource that was hugely influential for us in terms of learning how to soothe and settle Oria was the "Happiest Baby on The Block" book and DVD from Dr. Harvey Karp MD. At first I was not at all attracted to this work, as it seemed to have a very "commercial" appearance and I assumed that it was some mainstream baby book I'd have no interest in. However, after countless recommendations, I decided to check it out and was *soooooooooo* grateful that I did, especially once Oria was here.

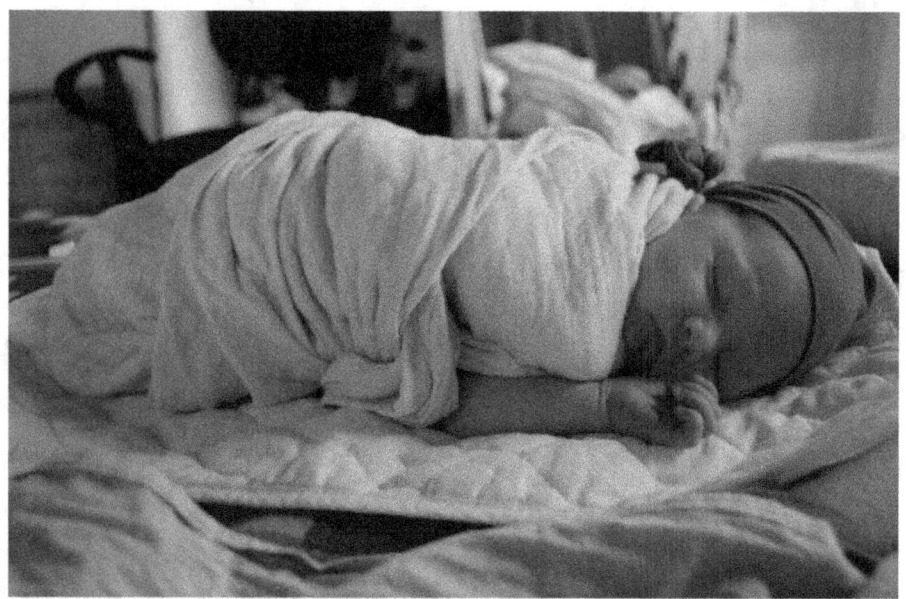

Dr. Karp shares five main ways to soothe distressed babies, especially those with "colic", however the techniques can help any baby. The techniques are to swaddle a baby, lay them on their side, make a loud "sshhhhhhhhhhhhh" noise in their ear (or any loud white noise), swing/rock/jiggle them rhythmically and give them something to suck on, like a nipple or finger. These soothing practices can help to emulate the womb environment for the baby and provide comfort. It may not be necessary to practice all five of these techniques simultaneously to soothe a baby though – sometimes one might work, or different techniques for different times/situations. Oria loves all five of these soothers. I felt especially grateful for learning about swaddling from this book and DVD. Swaddling a baby means to wrap them up tightly in a blanket, emulating the tight confines of the womb, keeping them warm and helping them to sleep snugly without startling themselves with their own jerking movements. We swaddled Oria a great deal in her first few weeks as she was much happier that way… I'm not sure how she would have got *any* sleep at that point without being swaddled – she would shock herself repeatedly with her flailing limbs whenever unwrapped… After four or five weeks she was getting better control over her movements and we started to put clothes on her more often, rather than swaddling her. As I write, we're at the stage where Oria is only swaddled for sleeping and wears clothes the rest of the time. I imagine that in another few weeks she'll probably not enjoy swaddling so much anymore, so we'll move on…for now she still sleeps so much better if swaddled.

Oria is also highly responsive to white noise in terms of soothing. She absolutely *loves* being near our stone-grinder nut butter machines, or the dehydrator, when either are running…she also likes audio tracks of ocean sounds or rain played at high volume…she responds well to loud "shhhhhhhhhhhhhhhhh"-ing in her ear too, or rhythmic "shhh-shhhhh-shhh"-ing… If she is in a phase of feeling soothed by one of these sounds and it suddenly stops, she immediately gets upset again.

The other soother that she loves is rhythmic bouncing/jiggling/swinging/rocking movements. This might involve us walking around holding her with a bouncing motion in our step, bouncing on a large yoga ball with her in our arms, swinging in a swing chair with her on our laps, or the ultimate sleep-inducer: going on a trip in the car ;) Similarly as with the white noises, if Oria is in the process of being soothed by some rhythmical movement and it stops, she gets immediately upset again…

A word of warning: don't be surprised if once you start bouncing/jiggling, you can't stop…on many occasions I have seen myself and others pass the baby over to someone else and still be bouncing around many minutes later, even though the baby is with someone else ;)

I feel extremely blessed to have all of these kinds of soothing tips available to us, especially for managing the first few weeks together and setting up a nice bond, so that Oria feels listened to, content and able to trust us to help her out when she is distressed.

I always like to keep in mind the phrase "if it ain't broken, don't try to fix it" in terms of soothing Oria; i.e. if I'm doing something to soothe her and it's *working*, it makes far more sense in my experience to just *stay* in that position/place, than to try out other soothing methods right then.

I'd also like to mention again here how *different* all babies are – what soothes one may be totally ineffective with another, plus each individual's preferences can change over time too. For example, people often seem to soothe babies off to sleep by singing lullabies…well, good luck trying that with Oria ;) There's no *way* this little girl would go off to sleep just from someone singing a song to her – not at this stage at least. Now, make a loud "shhhhhhhhh" noise in her ear though while she's swaddled in your arms next to the spinning stone-grinding machines and you might be on to something…

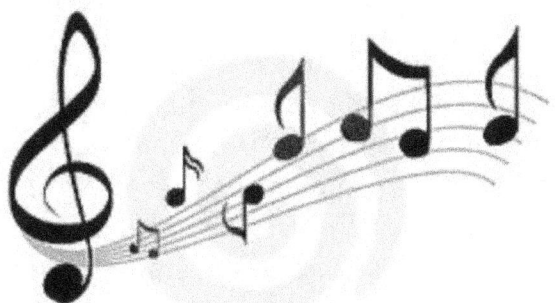

I think it's also very wise to be prepared in advance of the arrival of your little one with a selection of gentle, soothing, calming music to play in the background, either to help them with sleep or just to have playing in general. You might choose gentle classical music, sweet lullabies, whale/dolphin/ocean sounds or whatever feels good to you.

Water Baby

Oria was born into water and she seems to thoroughly enjoy being back in our huge bath every day for splashing, swimming and bathing joys. We are following the instructions from British baby swimming expert Lauren Heston to help Oria feel totally confident and competent in the water. Babies can swim long before they can usually crawl or walk, so it can be a wonderful gift to your little one to help them develop their water skills from the earliest possibility – literally from birth if you choose.

Baby Clothing

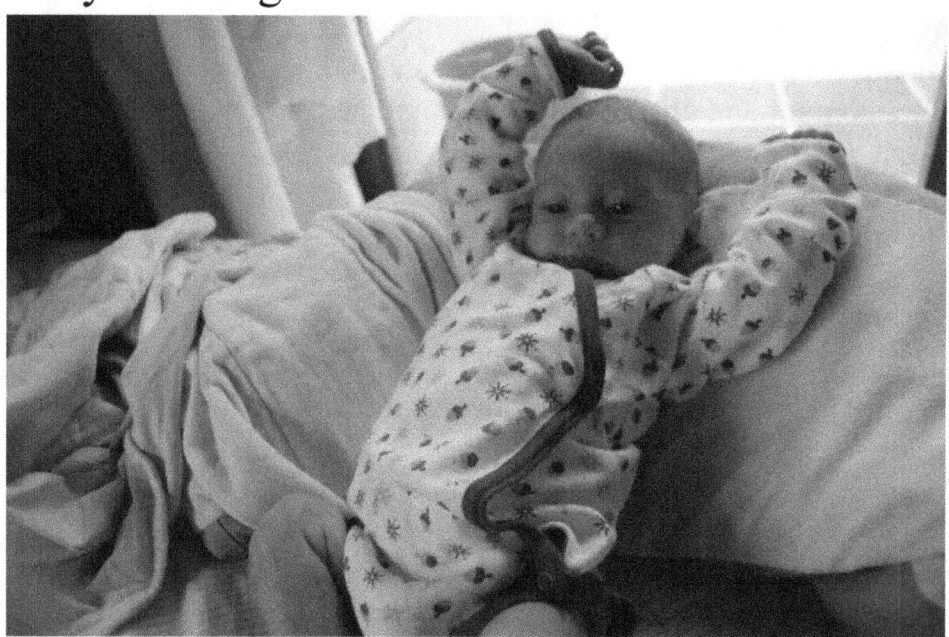

Where we live, in Ecuador, it's very challenging to find any "eco" clothing – nearly all clothing here is made from highly synthetic materials. So, in preparation for the arrival of our baby, we researched and bought all of her "eco"-clothing and other baby items online in the USA. In the first weeks of Oria's life, the items I found the most useful for her were muslin blankets, "pre-fold" nappy/diaper cloths, plus tiny socks, hats and mittens (to help her to stop cutting herself with tiny fingernails). As she got older, we moved on to using more of her clothes; the items we've so far loved best have been from the following companies: Kicky Pants (many gorgeous bamboo items: gowns, tops, hats, dresses), Under The Nile (great long-sleeved organic cotton tops), Bambinoland (organic cotton muslin blankets and thick, warm baby gowns), Baby Bambu (great little bamboo gowns) and Frugi in the UK (organic gowns, "onesies" and more…) I like the tiny little organic cotton socks from Ecoland best and we got many colourful pairs of organic cotton legwarmers too, from BabyLegs (great for doing Elimination Communication). I also appreciate the organic "SwaddleMe" sleep sacks - though we didn't have these in Oria's first weeks, they are great now for helping her get bundled up and off to sleep easily while she's still so young. She doesn't have any shoes yet, though many people have recommended "Robeez" shoes to us for babies and/or tiny moccasins.

Almost all of the clothing I bought for her in advance is green in colour, partly because it's my favourite colour and partly because we didn't know if a boy or a girl was coming to join us, so green seemed like a good neutral colour for either.

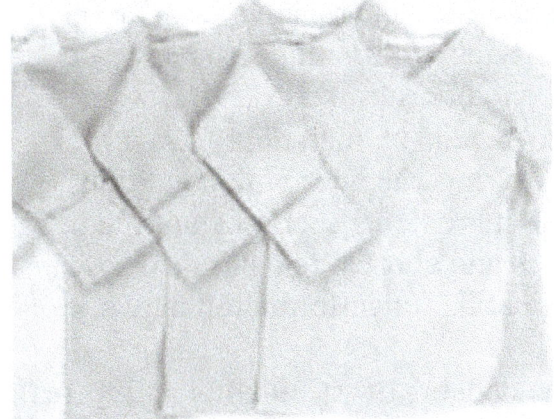

I was very happy to receive the guidance from one midwife friend to purchase clothing that is really easy to get on and off of babies, e.g. side openings rather than over-the-head openings, snap-fastenings rather than buttons and so on. This has proved to make dressing Oria a lot easier. I was also really excited to realise, when she'd been wearing clothes for a few weeks, that the items I *had* been putting on over her head could actually be put on her *feet-first* instead in almost all instances (many babies don't enjoy clothing going on over their heads).

Later in this book you can find a list of exactly what we bought in preparation for Oria's arrival and which items we found most useful.

Entertainment

If you're anything like me, around the two-month mark, you might be wondering how to *entertain* your baby between feeding/sleeping sessions. This is a kind of "in-between" stage, where your baby is no longer a tiny, floppy, sleepy newborn and yet they are also not yet at the stage of playing with things by themselves, or being able to even sit up for that matter. Other than simply having Oria with us as we went about our daily lives, here are some other examples of things we did/do to help keep her "entertained": making funny faces/noises/voices (human faces are usually a baby's favourite form of entertainment), doing daily massage, bathing/swimming/splashing in the bath daily, going for walks, reading books out loud to her, dancing with her, singing songs, showing her herself in a mirror, giving her some "tummy time" – laying her down on her belly with her hands positioned under her shoulders, to help strengthen her neck/back muscles, showing her different things such as crystals/paintings etc and talking about them, putting simple toys like the Skwish wooden toy in her hands to look at, or a little rattle and so on… Little babies are like sponges – they're interested in seemingly just about *anything*, especially in terms of understanding what it means to be an adult human here, so have fun showing them the world :)

Unvaccinated

Like many "natural"-minded parents, we choose not to give Oria any vaccinations. We choose instead to do the best we can to support her own immune system to be strong and healthy, especially through colostrum and breastmilk.

There are myriad reasons why we don't choose to vaccinate, including: it's completely unnatural, there's abundant evidence linking vaccines with conditions such as autism/ADHD, vaccines have highly toxic ingredients such as aluminium, anti-freeze, formaldehyde, mercury, animal viruses and aborted fetus tissue and we have no desire to be part of the fear-driven, intimidating, misinformation network of western medicine.

The website vacinfo.org has masses of info on the dangers of vaccination and a great slogan too: "educate before you vaccinate". The website is headed up by speaker April Renee, whose own 4-year-old daughter died from vaccination poisoning some years ago. Anti-vaccination campaigner Jock Doubleday also has a long-standing vaccine challenge on the go, wherein he is offering over $250,000 to any doctor or pharmaceutical CEO willing to drink a vaccine cocktail. This offer has been valid for over a decade already at the time of writing and no-one has ever taken Jock up on the challenge – rather revealing…

Food and Medicines

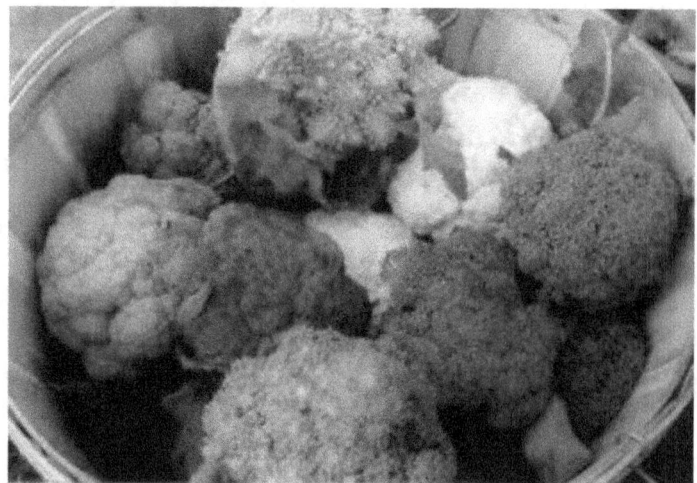

There are many foods that breastfeeding mothers are not advised to consume, to help make digestion easier for the baby. These foods include garlic, onions, all

70

"brassica/cruciferous" veggies like kale, broccoli, cabbage etc, spicy foods, orange juice, dairy and more… One raw friend told me that she pretty much just ate simple salads and drank juices for the first six months or so of life with her two children, as this helped greatly to reduce digestive issues with the babies and helped the whole family get more rest and sleep. I am pretty much excluding all of those listed things from my intake too, though I may have a small amount of kale/garlic/spice here and there – I certainly don't make these items a key part of my intake though at this point. You may feel somewhat "limited" in terms of food choices in these first months, however, remember that it's all in the interests of making life easier for both you and the baby, which is surely worth it in the long-run. As they get older, babies' digestive systems get stronger, plus they are more ready for solids and experimentation, so you can explore more in the culinary world again then too…

On the subject of eating *raw* while breastfeeding, please note that it might be quite tricky for you to use a high-speed blender anymore to make smoothies and so on, if you are "baby-wearing" your little one, as these machines can be extremely loud and hurt baby's ears. You may want to ask other people for help blending, or prepare everything, place baby far away and blend, or get one of the special plastic casings for blenders that are used commercially to reduce noise in cafes and so on. Smoothies can be such a great, fast, nourishing water-rich meal choice for new mamas, yet it's not a practical choice if you can't easily use a blender, so you might want to find a solution for this in advance…

Personally I still eat totally raw vegan/"bee-gan" post-partum and am feeling great. I pretty much each just as I did pre-pregnancy and through pregnancy; nothing has really changed, other than now avoiding those foods listed here that aren't so helpful while breastfeeding. I have no intention to eat any other way at present.

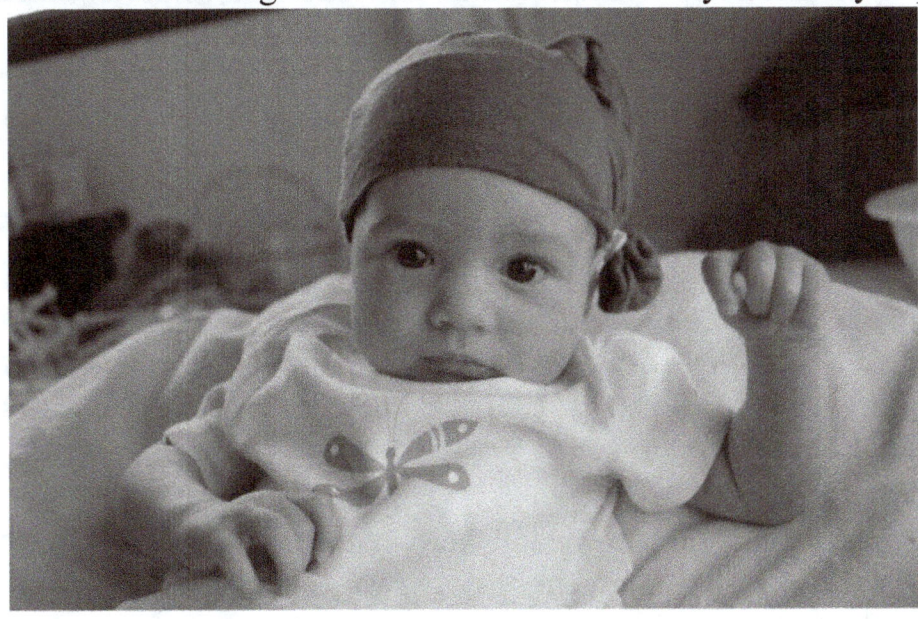

It is our intention to raise Oria eating in the same way that we do: raw vegan/"bee-gan", however, I am of course open to incorporating other things for her like raw dairy/eggs, for example, if it seems like this is what would serve her best and she likes it. I am also very aware that as she grows up, she's likely to want to try other kinds of foods. It is not my intention to try to restrict any experimentation she might seek, as I strongly suspect that ultimately she will gravitate back to eating in whichever way feels best to her.

Also, as a result of her healthy upbringing, with "food being her medicine and medicine her food", it is my hope that Oria will encounter minimal illness along her journey…if for some reason she *is* dealing with some illness, it would certainly be our intention to help treat her with natural, "alternative" solutions such as herbal medicine, homoeopathy, energy medicine and so on. Of course in the case of any acute/emergency situation, such as her breaking a bone, for example, we would surely seek "western" medical help, however otherwise we aim to keep away from mainstream western doctors, hospitals and medicines.

Baby Burping

I have come to believe that it is a very wise practice for babies to be "burped" after each and every feeding. We learnt this the hard way… We did *some* burping of Oria here and there in her first few weeks, nothing consistent though, until we heard the recommendation to burp babies consistently after every feeding, so that gas doesn't build up so much in their systems all day and cause them grief by the evening time… We had been going through a phase of Oria crying in the evenings (not full-on "colic", yet not fun for anyone to experience), so we started to practice this idea of consistent burping after every meal and it seemed to help her out a lot. Hence I would highly recommend for any other new parents to get into the habit of consistently "burping" your baby as often as you can… One friend told me that she was advised by her midwife to always aim for getting four burps out at least, at each burping, as a general guideline.

For those who are unfamiliar, "burping" a baby usually involves holding them in an upright position of some kind – maybe up against your shoulder, or sitting upright, or being held upright in some other way (some babies also seem to do well draped belly-down across a caregiver's thighs). You might pat/rub the baby's back, jiggle them gently or rock them, anything to help the little air bubbles in their bellies bubble up to the top and release…and remember that just as with adults, the burps may not always be very loud or even audible.

Enjoy Every Moment

After Oria's birth, one of the main comments people kept sharing with us over and over and *over* again was to "enjoy every moment, they grow up so fast". We literally heard or read this *hundreds* of times over from different people, so it seemed worth paying attention to… We feel very blessed to be able to receive insights from so many people around the world, as it gives us a great overview of what might be wise to pay attention to… Hearing this "enjoy every moment" comment *so* many times over helped remind us to stay present with Oria and do our best to make the most of every moment of every day with her. Remember that you have the possibility to drop the story and just be here now - this present moment is the only thing you really have and you will never have it again, so enjoy.

Another comment we repeatedly hear from other parents is that "it gets better all the time". Well, we're excited to see how that keeps on unfolding from here… ;)

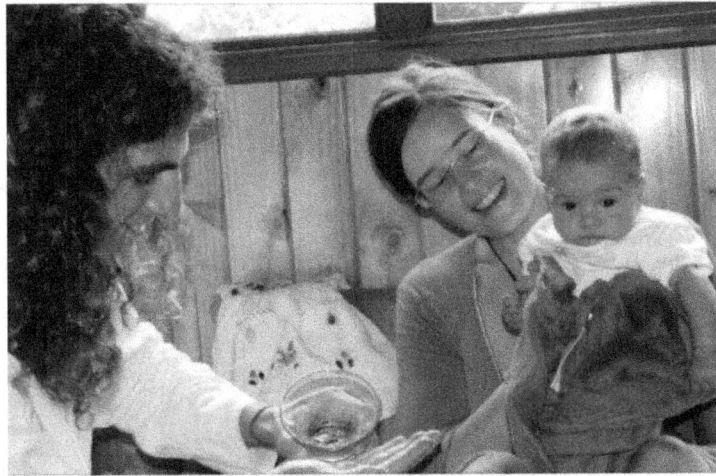

Blessingway

A rite of passage that we were excited to share with Oria was a "Blessingway" gathering, which we held on the day that she turned three months of age. We gathered in circle that day with like-minded, loving friends and asked each person who was willing, to share with us something for our journey onwards here together as a family – perhaps some sage guidance, perhaps a song, a poem, a story, a dance or whatever came to mind.

We gathered many small pieces of quartz crystal from our land prior to the event and set them to charge in Oria's energy field for a week leading up to the Blessingway, then we gifted a piece of this quartz to each person at the gathering. We conducted a beautiful water ceremony for Oria too, anointing her with water that had been blessed by the whole group and even charged with a piece of marble from Osho himself. Mr. M and I also drank some of this charged water and we poured the rest over the bowl of quartz crystals to energise them further.

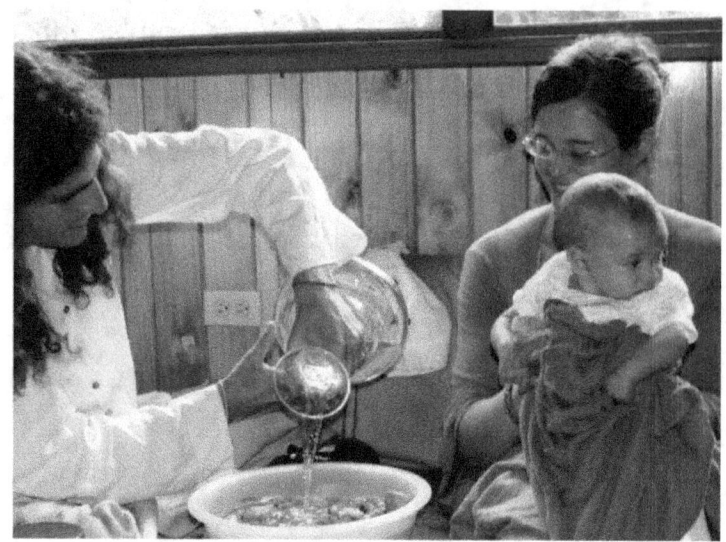

Three months seemed like a nice milestone for such a gathering to me, as it marked the end of the so-called "fourth trimester", when the baby starts to usually be less "fetus-like" and dependent. We also chose to touch Oria's feet directly to the ground that day too, to mark her full embodiment here on Earth. As far as I know, she had not yet directly touched the ground herself up until that point, though she had been and still is regularly grounded via grounding pads in our house and through being in the arms of other people who are grounded.

Oria's Blessingway was a beautiful, loving, heart-filling day of celebration with wonderful people and the memories from this celebration will surely stay with us for life. I'd highly recommend such a ceremony for anyone else interested in honouring their baby's journey here in such a way.

The Three Month Tipping Point

For us, it was really fascinating to note how Oria seemed to go through some significant shifts immediately after turning three months of age. It was truly like she hit the end of that "fourth trimester" and suddenly started showing up quite differently. She seemed to suddenly be so much more present, aware and engaged in life, she became even more vocal with her attempts to speak and (blessedly), the evening crying bouts pretty much abruptly ceased…very interesting and we feel very grateful ;)

Our Intentions for The Future

As I write this, Oria has been here Earthside just a few months, yet I would love to share here some of our intentions for life with this precious little button as it unfolds from here...

Unschooling

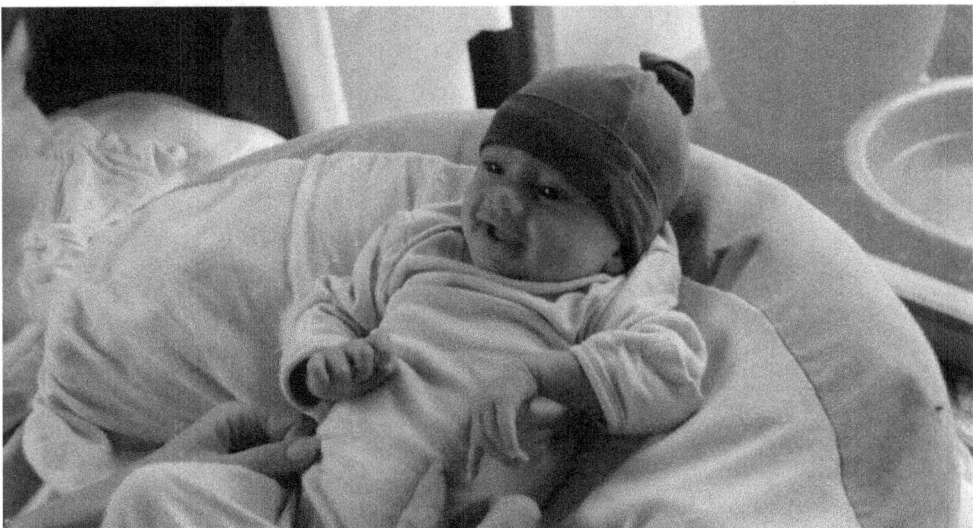

It is our intention to "unschool" with Oria, meaning that she will go about life with us, learning from everyday experiences and pursuing the things that *she* is interested in, rather than being subjected to any curriculums or formal schooling systems. It would be my personal hope for her that she gets to learn lots of useful, practical life skills like gardening, foraging, childcare, house building and so on... I would hope too that there is at least one musical instrument she loves to play... We have no attachments though to how her path unfolds and choose simply to support whatever unfolds for her in terms of her interests.

I'm also excited for Oria that she gets to grow up bilingual here in Ecuador, hearing English and Spanish daily. *(I am also speaking Icelandic to her, though I'm not fluent, so I'm not sure she's going to end up speaking great Icelandic if she only hears me – I'm always excited to see if other Icelandic speakers may end up in this area at some point... ;)*

Non-Violent/Compassionate Communication

I am a HUGE fan of Non-Violent Communication (NVC, also often referred to as "Compassionate Communication"). If you're not familiar with this wonderful system for connecting with others with compassion and love, you might like to see the book "Non-Violent Communication" by Marshall Rosenburg, or the main NVC website at www.cnvc.org. It is my desire and intention to practice NVC-style communication with Oria to the best of my abilities as she grows up with us. Author Naomi Aldort has some GREAT ideas along these lines in her book "Raising Our Children, Raising Ourselves." Some of the ideas that really resonate for me include: treating the child as an "equal" in the sense of respecting that they are an individual with preferences and choices to be made, rather than trying to "control" them or order them around; treating the child in the way one might treat a valued guest in your home; helping the child to trust their own feelings and intuition; choosing to always support and validate the child, like a really good friend, rather than "betraying" them around others by belittling them, revealing their secrets/concerns or allowing others to speak to them in ways that the child finds uncomfortable, without supporting the child to feel respected.

I have long had a little saying in my life in regards to relationships that has steered me well: "feelings first". If someone around me seems to be upset/uncomfortable/exuberant/angry or experiencing any other strong emotion that they want to express and share about, *this* is what comes first, rather than anything else that I might *think* I want to give my attention to…in my experience, if I take the time to put feelings first, hear the other person out (or express the feelings myself if it is me with the strong emotional field), then the feelings can be honoured and can pass much more smoothly. If, instead, something else is prioritised ahead of the feelings being expressed, this can lead to further complications and even eruptions, in my experience…so, my preference is definitely to aim to put "feelings first" in communication.

I also like to remember the fact that, all being well, I am going to share a lot more of life with Oria with her as an *adult*, rather than as a child, so if I can do my best to communicate with her while she is a child with compassion, love and grace, we have a much stronger chance to share a strong, loving, mutually respectful connection when she is older.

Media and Other External Influences

It is our intention to bring Oria up with as little influence from the "mainstream" media as possible. Neither Mr. M or I have watched television for at least a decade at the time of writing, so TV is definitely not something we're excited to share with her, in fact there is not even a TV in our house…

We don't have any magazines or newspapers around, no smartphones or radio and there are also very few billboards around in the countryside here in Ecuador. We play music that we love, have many lovely books around and occasionally watch a carefully selected film for entertainment (e.g. no or minimal violence/swearing/scary behaviour). It would be our intention to continue in this vein now that Oria is here with us…we also do not intend to expose her to mainstream children's entertainment such as Disney films, children's music, computer games and plastic toys. We have some lovely, co-operation-based board games here for when she is older and a whole world of natural wonders to explore outside in our gardens, orchards and forests. We also have fun outside amenities available such as a trampoline, swimming pool, basketball/tennis court, hiking paths and so on.

I imagine that the internet/computers *will* be part of Oria's life, as this is a big part of our own lives and the internet can be such a rich, useful resource, easy to tailor to one's own interests/preferences. I imagine that at some stage we may want to establish some boundaries in terms of what Oria looks at online and for how long…I guess we'll cross such bridges if and when we come to them… ;)

Personally, I am excited to see who this little girl becomes, without the influence of "civilised" mainstream Western media all around her…

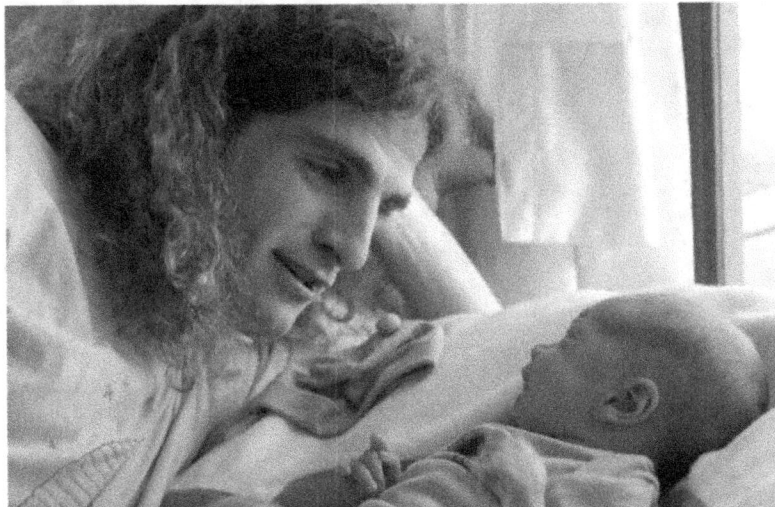

Different Styles

I'd love to highlight the idea that different caretakers for a child may have rather different "styles" in terms of how they are with the child and it might be in everyone's highest interest for you to be *relaxed* with this reality, rather than trying to get someone else to treat the child exactly as you do. It seems common, for example, for mamas to get upset with their partners for behaving differently with the baby than they would. The mother is usually the one who is with the child most of the time, so she may get a little "rigid" in her head that *her* way of doing things with the baby is "the" way to do things. While it can of course be true that she likely has some great insights into what works and doesn't work well with the child, it's also possible that her partner has unique insights and ways of connecting with the child too. The child can experience a *mix* of caretaking styles, games and ways of being, rather than everything feeling uniform with every person. As an example, a friend of mine has a son who he sees at weekends, as he and the boy's mother are separated. Whereas the mother provides a very solid, stable, grounded, secure environment for the lad, his father provides a much more "adventurous", colourful, free-flowing environment. The boy gets to experience and enjoy both of these very different parenting styles and neither is "right" or "wrong", they're just different. The same can be allowed to flow in contexts where the parents or caregivers are together, as long as each person is open and allowing of each other's care-giving styles.

Baby Shopping

When I started to investigate, pre-pregnancy, exactly what we might love to have on hand for the arrival of a child, I was horrified…there were *sooooooooooo* many things available in the baby realm. I found it completely overwhelming at first and didn't know where to start. I knew it couldn't be *this* complicated, so I started asking other "eco" minded mums and midwives what they actually found useful to have in the first year of a little one's life and made myself a master list based on those recommendations. Here below is the list of what I purchased in preparation *(remember, we live in Ecuador, where "eco"-anything is in short supply, so I was preparing clothing etc for the whole first year, to have everything here on hand.)*

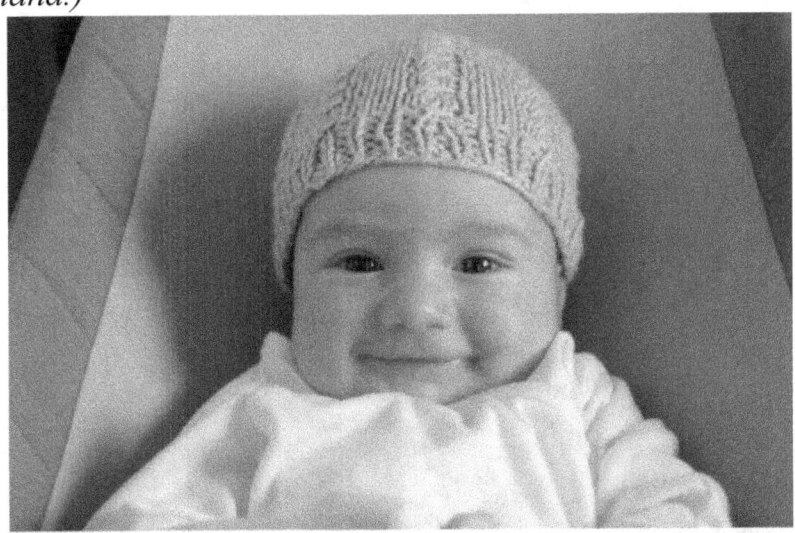

Let's also be clear that tiny babies truly have very few wants in terms of physical goods – they pretty much want to be held in a warm loving embrace with a nipple available to feed from…anything else beyond that is somewhat superlative to a baby's personal desires…they don't come in expecting to find a wipes warmer, a playmat, crib, hanging mobile, selection of cuddly toys and so on… ;) *We* might find it easier to have certain things available for our parenting journey – the baby is likely to be indifferent to these choices though, at least in the very beginning…

You'll notice in the lists below that I got some items for cloth diapering – though we are practicing EC with Oria, we wanted to have *some* items on hand for cloth diapering in case of trips, being in unfamiliar places and so on. If you intend to fully practice cloth diapering and not EC, I imagine you'd want many more supplies than the amounts listed here…

I also found it somewhat odd while I was accumulating all of these supplies that I basically seemed to be acquiring a huge amount of *fabric* in lots of different shapes and sizes – this piece is for this purpose, that piece is used for that…it's all just fabric… It brought a whole new meaning for me of bringing a child into the "material" world ;) So I strongly suspect that if you are even slightly talented with a sewing machine, you could create a lot of baby supplies for yourself, armed with just a long stretch of organic cotton and some threads…

I bought almost everything for Oria from Amazon.com, as it's easy to find a huge range of items there, the prices are usually very good and their service is very efficient in my experience. They also have a wonderful programme called "Amazon Mom" which I would definitely recommend joining. The "Amazon Mom" service is free to join and brings many benefits, including free "Prime" 2-day shipping, special baby-related deals every week, exclusive discounts and more – you can join here: http://www.amazon.com/gp/mom/signup/info *(though sometimes there is a waiting list to join)*. I also bought some things directly from bambinoland.com (muslin blankets, thick organic blankets and kimonos) and etsy.com (handmade items like cloth menstrual pads, chime necklaces).

I have done my best to hyperlink every product here to a place where you can find that item for purchase online – please note however that product availability can change over time. Also, in instances where there are multiple items listed together, e.g. "18 muslin blankets", I have hyperlinked that name to my *favourite* example of those products.

(This list includes extra muslin/receiving blankets that people gifted us after Oria's birth, plus "SwaddleMe" wraps and extra waterproof-backed change pads that we bought after birth.)

24 simple organic cotton "pre-fold" nappies/diapers

3 extra organic "pre-folds" from Babykicks

3 large hemp "all-in-one" nappies/diapers

2 small hemp "all-in-one" nappies/diapers

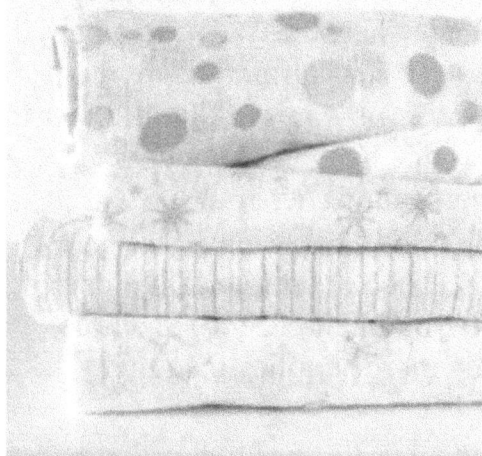

20 organic cotton breastpads (from different companies)

10 organic "nursing" bras – different styles, sizes, colours (my favourites are from Majamas)

40 "burp cloths" from different companies

8 waterproof plastic nappy/diaper covers, 4 smaller, 4 larger

waterproof nappy/diaper bag

organic sling/pouch

2 organic Moby wraps (to always have one available, when the other is being washed)

18 muslin blankets

14 receiving blankets – different materials, colours, styles

5 "SwaddleMe" wraps

12 waterproof-backed organic cotton change pads

3 toys – cherry wood rattle, wooden Manhattan Skwish toy, Sophie the Giraffe natural rubber teething toy

Boba organic baby carrier

Blessed Nest breastfeeding pillow

Babybjorn baby potty

Babybjorn organic bouncing chair

Gliding chair

Bob pushchair/stroller

Pack of 5 Snappi bungees

Natural Nipple Butter from Earth Mama Angel Baby

Various baby bottom balms

Jai Baby Joy massage oil

Andreas' White Sesame Oil

Sitz bath herbs

Stethoscope

Thermometer

Baby nail clippers

Plastic sheets for beds (these go underneath usual sheets, to stop any "accidents" seeping through into mattress.)

Surgical scissors

Umbilical cord clamp

Bulb syringe

Amber teething necklace

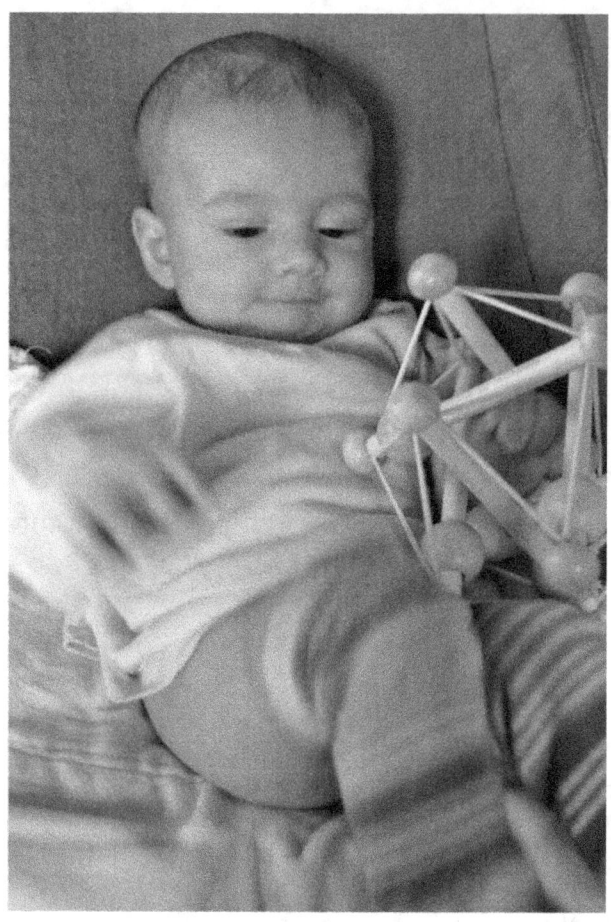

People have also gifted us soft toys and children's books for Oria since her birth – she doesn't show much *interest in either yet, though I'm sure she will in time...*

Clothes 0-3 months (This list includes clothing items that people gifted us after Oria's birth)

3 pairs socks

8 pairs legwarmers

4 little hats

2 little sunhats

9 gowns – different colours/materials (elasticated at the end, easier to get on and off baby, especially when practicing EC)

1 all-in-one "romper suit"

3 short-sleeved t-shirts

5 long-sleeved t-shirts

4 "onesies"

1 Lana Care wool long-sleeved top

2 tiny swimming costumes (bathing suits)

2 pairs tiny mittens

Clothes 3-6 months

3 pairs socks
1 t-shirt
1 long-sleeved t-shirt
1 swing dress
1 gown

Clothes 6-9 months

1 hat
3 t-shirts
4 long-sleeved t-shirts
2 onesies
3 pairs of leggings/trousers

Clothes 9-12 months

1 hat
8 short-sleeved onesies
2 long-sleeved gowns

Herbs:

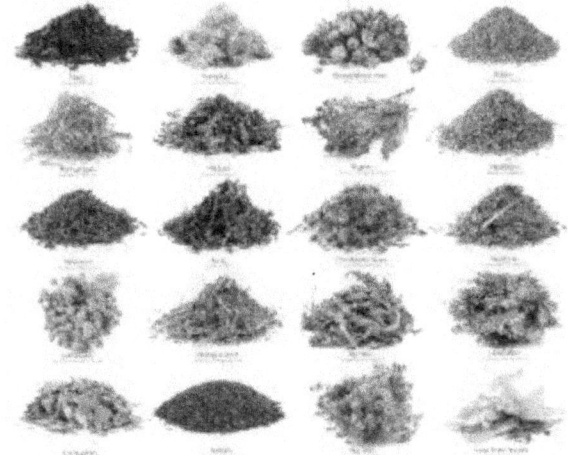

I ordered a *mass* of dried/tinctured herbs from MountainRoseHerbs.com in preparation for pregnancy, birth and life immediately post-partum. I made my choices based almost solely on the recommendations in Susun Weed's fabulous book "Wild Woman Herbal for the Childbearing Year". This is what I acquired, listed with dried herbs first, followed by tinctures (extracts):

Wild Yam Root
Witch Hazel Leaf
Cramp Bark

Red Clover Herb
Raspberry Leaf
Nettle Leaf
Angelica Root powder
Anise Seed powder
Fennel Seed
Peppermint Leaf
Spearmint
Black Haw Bark
Dandelion Leaf
Yellow Dock Root
Comfrey Leaf
Blue Cohosh Root Powder
Witch Hazel Bark powder
Partridgeberry Herb
Motherwort extract
Echinacea Purpurea extract
Blessed Thistle extract
Angelica extract
Shepherd's Purse extract
Skullcap extract
Wild Yam extract

Things we use daily that we already had:

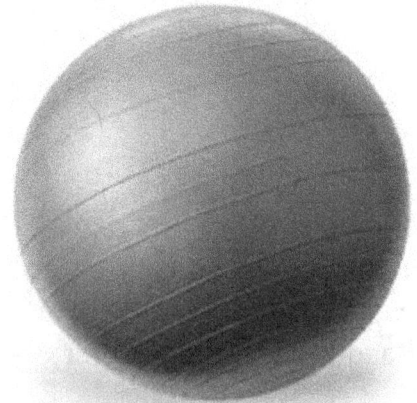

Plastic box with lid (for catching EC deposits)
My bamboo clothing
Flip camera and photo camera for recording precious moments

Yoga ball

Pillows (stacked into the wall next to our bed, so I can lean back into them to breastfeed comfortably)

Bath

Salt lamp

EMF protectors (to help shield Oria and us from EMFs)

Stone-grinders (for white noise – you could also use a washing machine, white noise machine/CD, hairdryer etc)

Usefulness…

I'd love to further share here how *useful* we found each of these items, as perhaps it might help other new parents to work out what may be truly useful with a new baby. I have divided up all of the items above into things we found either extremely useful, pretty useful or those that we've barely/never used:

Here are the items we find extremely useful:

-"Pre-fold" nappies/diapers

-Burp cloths (I like the ones from the "Babykicks" company best)

-2 organic Moby wraps

-Muslin blankets

-Receiving blankets

-Waterproof-backed organic cotton change pads

-Blessed Nest breastfeeding pillow

-All clothing 0-3 months and some clothing 3-6 months

-Natural Nipple Butter (I actually used less than one pot of this in the end)

-Baby Bottom Balm from Earth Mama Angel Baby

-Andreas' White Sesame Oil

-Plastic sheets for beds

-Herbs

-Plastic box with lid (for catching EC deposits)

-My bamboo clothing

-Flip camera and photo camera for recording precious moments

-Yoga ball

-Pillows

Plus all the items we use daily that we already had, e.g. bath, salt lamp, EMF protectors, stone-grinders for white noise, etc.

These are the things we've found pretty useful:
-Organic sling/pouch (seemed too precarious at first, more useful now that she has head control)
-Jai Baby Joy massage oil
-Babybjorn organic bouncing chair (we use it for her to sit in when we have no hands free and she wants to be upright)

These things we've either barely used so far or not used at all:
-"All-in-one" nappies/diapers
-Breastpads (I just caught the initial breastmilk overflow in a little bowl)
-Plastic nappy/diaper covers
-Waterproof nappy/diaper bag (just use on trips)
-Toys (she's not really interested in them yet)
-Boba organic baby carrier (this is for older babies)
-Babybjorn baby potty (using a plastic tub with lid so far)
-Gliding chair (I simply don't yet have this here – it's in the USA still as I write, or I would surely be sitting in it right now
-Bob pushchair/stroller (for when she's much older and getting trickier to carry)
-Most clothing 3-12 months (too big for now…)
-Pack of 5 Snappi bungees
-Sitz bath herbs (used aloe filets instead)
-Stethoscope
-Thermometer
-Baby nail clippers

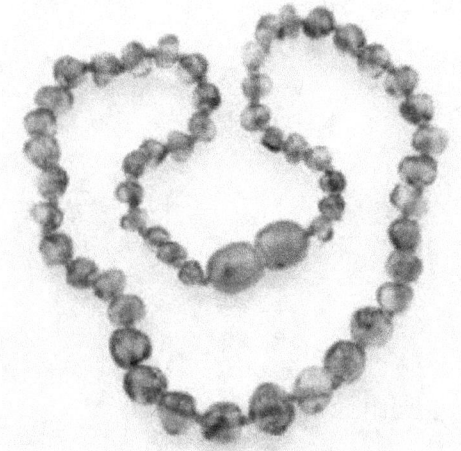

-Surgical scissors (to cut umbilical cord – didn't use)
-Umbilical cord clamp

-Bulb syringe (*essential* though, when we did use it, to clear mucus from Oria's mouth/nose at birth)

-Amber teething necklace (not needed yet)

Other Items

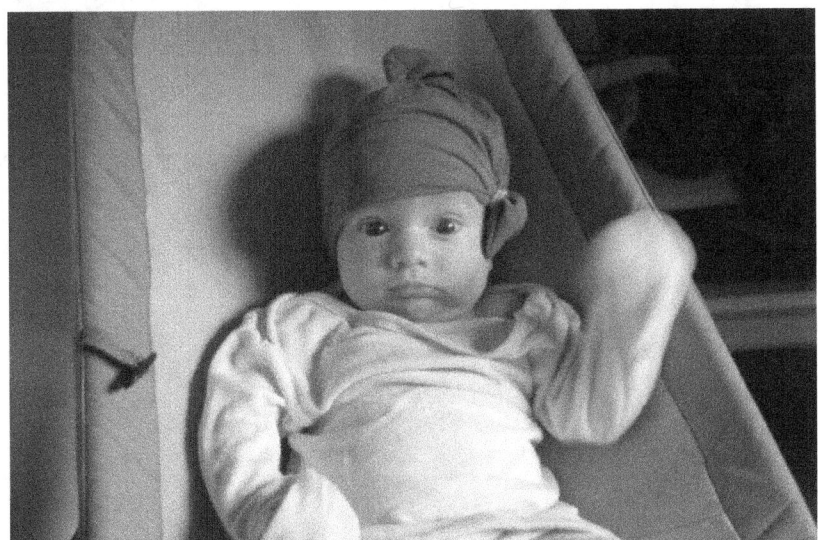

I thought it would also be useful to list here in one place other items mentioned in this book that you might love to have on hand, ready for the arrival of a little one. These are in no particular order…

-Thick menstrual pads
-Pregnancy test
-Enema bag
-Chime necklace
-"Baby and Me" pre-natal whole food tablets from Megafood
-Omega-Zen-3 (for DHA)
-Vitamin B12 patches
-Vitamin K2 caps
-Vitamin D spray
-Non-GMO lecithin powder (for choline, for brain development)
-Andreas' oils
-Bone Response/Bone Renewal
-Natural Calm
-Angstrom minerals of Zinc, Calcium, Iron
-Kelp capsules
-Rescue Remedy (in case of shock post-birth)
-Tahini

-Aloe vera leaves

-Coconuts/coconut water

-Colloidal Silver

-Algaes, like chlorella, spirulina and marine phytoplankton

-Herbs, such as: catnip, chamomile, fennel, lemon balm, red clover, peppermint, dill, anise, cumin, caraway, raspberry leaves, nettles, alfalfa, red clover, borage leaves, fenugreek, blessed thistle tincture, skullcap tincture, echinacea tincture (to stop infections)

-Supplies for lotus birth: salt, pungent dried herbs such as rosemary, lavender, nutmeg; something to hold the placenta like a thick cloth or little basket; encapsulation device and capsules to encapsulate dried placenta

Recommended Resources:

Books:

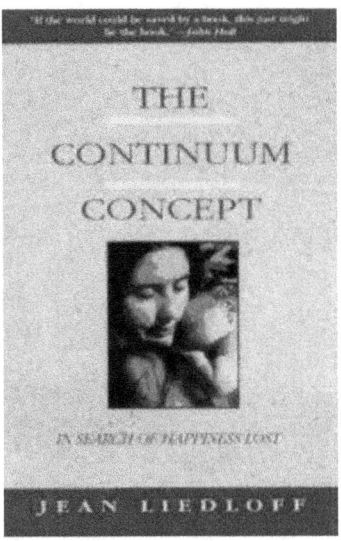

These are books that I have read and recommend, in alphabetical order by book name, with my favourites asterixed (*):

"After The Baby's Birth" by Robin Lim*

"Anastasia" by Vladimir Megre (and the whole "Ringing Cedars" book series)*

"Birthing From Within" by Pam England and Rob Horowitz

"Birthkeepers" by Veronika Robinson*

"Continuum Concept" by Jean Liedloff*

"Diaper-Free" by Ingrid Bauer*

"Evie's Kitchen" by Shazzie*

"Gentle Birth Choices" by Barbara Harper

"Gentle Birth, Gentle Mothering" by Dr. Sarah Buckley*

"Ina May's Guide to Childbirth" by Ina May Gaskin*

"Ina May's Guide to Breastfeeding" by Ina May Gaskin*

"Placenta" by Robin Lim*

"Raising Our Children, Raising Ourselves" by Naomi Aldort*

"Spiritual Midwifery" by Ina May Gaskin*

"The Drinks Are On Me" by Veronika Robinson*

"The Happiest Baby On The Block" by Dr. Harvey Karp, M.D.*

"Unassisted Childbirth" by Laura Shanley*

"What Mothers Do: Especially When It Looks Like Nothing" by Naomi Stadlen*

"Wise Woman Herbal for The Child-Bearing Year" by Susun Weed*

Other books that I own but didn't get to read yet:
"Birth Matters" by Ina May Gaskin
"Childbirth Without Fear" by Grantly Dick-Read
"How To Talk So Kids Will Listen And Listen So Kids Will Talk" by Adele Faber and Elaine Mazlish
"Hygieia: A Woman's Herbal" by Jeannine Parvati Baker
"Magical Child" by Joseph Chilton Pearce
"Parenting From Your Heart" by Inbal Kashtan
"Respectful Parents, Respectful Kids" by Sura Hart and Victoria Kindle Hodson
"The Baby Signing Book" by Sara Bingham
"The Natural Child" by Jan Hunt

DVDs that we love:

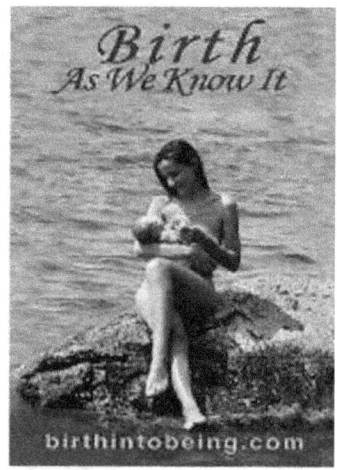

"Babies"
"Birth As We Know It"/"Birth Into Being"
"Dunstan Baby Language"
"Orgasmic Birth"
"The Happiest Baby On The Block"
"Waterbabies"

Other useful resources:

*ConsciousParentingSummit.com – check out this amazing set of audio interviews we conducted with a group of many of the most influential people in the "Conscious

Parenting" realm, including: Sarah Buckley, MD, Robin Lim, Ingrid Bauer, Elena Vladirimova, Naomi Aldort, Laura Shanley, April Renee, Barbara Harper, Shazzie and many others.

*I'd *highly* recommend attending a "birthshop" with gentle birth legend Elena Vladirimova – see http://birthintobeing.com - we attended one of her weekend classes a couple of years before conceiving and it was extremely influential for us.

*"The Mother" magazine – this fabulous, long-running magazine on "natural" parenting themes is key reading for those interested in this way of life. I regularly gift subscriptions for this magazine to pregnant friends, as I think it's such a great resource. See themothermagazine.co.uk (British site) or themothermagazine.org (N. American site) to subscribe.

*PositiveBirthStories.com – this was one of very few sites online that I found with *positive* birthing stories to share.

*I also liked to poke around on YouTube using search terms like "unassisted birth", "water birth", "lotus birth" and so on, to see inspiring stories. As the saying goes "a picture is worth a thousand words" and actually *seeing* other women giving birth easily, ecstatically, even *orgasmically*, can help make a great impact on your mind and help undo any previous fear-based programming…

*BreastfeedingInc.ca - Dr. Jack Newman's site, with GREAT little free videos showing how to successfully breastfeed.

*ttfuture.org/authors/jleidloff – this link takes you to a fabulous, highly insightful hour-long, free video interview with the late Jean Liedloff, author of "The Continuum Concept".

*babycenter.com – I found a lot of very useful, practical information on this site, despite the fact that it looks very "commercial". It seems to be one of the largest baby websites online and comes up frequently when I search for things on Google.

*BlessYouMom.com – I love the beautiful card decks of affirmative slogans for mums from this site.

*I appreciate a lot of the lovely organic herbal teas from Earth Mama Angel Baby too, such as "Morning Wellness" tea, "Third Trimester" tea and "Milkmaid Tea". You can check out all of their fabulous goodies at earthmamaangelbaby.com.

*hm4hb.net - a friend recently told me about the fabulous worldwide "Human Milk for Human Babies" groups. This grass-roots movement involves people all over the world providing extra human breastmilk to other people who could use more to feed their babies – hurray :)

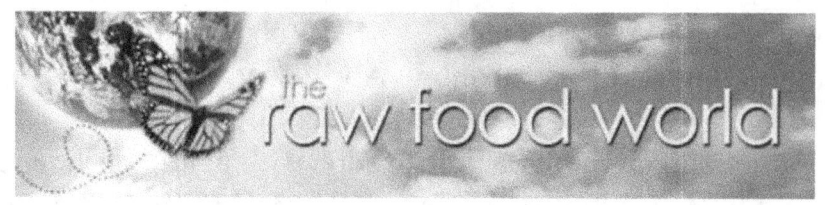

In our online store, www.TheRawFoodWorld.com, we sell many of the items mentioned in this book, such as: supplements, tahini, Natural Calm, books, DVDs, herbs, lecithin, Andreas' oils, enema bags and much more – check us out :)

You can also see videos and updates about our dear little daughter Oria on our blog: www.TheRawFoodWorld.tv.

Brightest blessings to everyone, for a gentle start :)

www.ingramcontent.com/pod-product-compliance
Lightning Source LLC
Chambersburg PA
CBHW080324290526
45793CB00006B/1199